CEU = 0.7

BAD
BLOOD

BAD BLOOD

CRISIS IN THE AMERICAN RED CROSS

JUDITH REITMAN

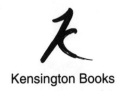

Kensington Books

KENSINGTON BOOKS are published by

Kensington Publishing Corp.
850 Third Avenue
New York, NY 10022

Library of Congress Card Catalog Number: 96-076491
ISBN 1-57566-115-2

First Printing: November, 1996
10 9 8 7 6 5 4 3 2 1

Printed in the United States of America

To my parents

TABLE OF CONTENTS

ACKNOWLEDGMENTS

The writing of BAD BLOOD was both intellectually and emotion-
ally demanding. As much as it was an investigative work, BAD
BLOOD became a metaphorical journey. Along the way, I found
many guides, people whose sense of conscience and justice opened
many doors.

This book owes its existence to my agent Deborah Schneider who
immediately recognized the importance of this story; Walter Zachar-
ius, Founder and Chairman of the Board of Kensington Books who
had the courage to publish this book; and Paul Dinas, Kensington's
editor-in-chief, who nurtured me and this project from conception
to completion. My family was, as always, a wellspring of support and
encouragement. The masterful research skills of Suzanne Roy, whose
patience was matched only by her tenacity, gave this book authority
and depth. My editorial colleague in London, Christine Murdock
kept me focused on the central issues. Years ago, Dr. Jan Moor-
Jankowski urged me to explore the issue of tainted blood and has
always been my enthusiastic supporter.

Of the many attorneys on whom I relied, Ashcraft & Gerel's Mike
Feldman, Chris Tisi and Peter Vangsnes's passionate involvement in
transfusion AIDS spurred me on to a deeper understanding of this
issue and directed me to individuals of courage and compassion,

principal among them Dr. Edgar Engleman and Dr. Don Francis. Steve Choquette of Holland & Hart spent innumerable instructional hours on the cases he tried. As always my attorney Philip Byler gave me wise counsel and advice and reminded me of the tenents of the First Amendment. Jim MacPherson of the Council of Community Blood Centers shared his invaluable perspective as did dozens of longtime blood banking officials.

I am profoundly grateful to the Michaels*, Ray, and Kirby families for welcoming me into their hearts and homes. Their lives are testament to the resiliency of the human spirit.

Thank yous to Carmen Santiago for the lessons in faith, to Vicki Ward who showed me that truth is rewarded, to Meredy van Syckle for the 'bigger picture,' Mary Ann and Lynn for the universal connection, and the cheering gallery at the Mayflower: Ken Sperry, Joel Levine, John Payne, David Smolover, and Kirsten Peckerman—all of whom kept me on track. Dimitri Rimsky for creative conduits, Karin Adams whose expert transcription went beyond the call of duty, Derek St. Pierre for research access, Louise Poletto, for the energizing and Molly Barnes for the nourishment. And, of course, Michelle Leigh for her worldly optimism. Thank you, too, to Cyndy Brissett for her doggedness. Special thanks to Katherine Gayle for her cheerful editorial assistance.

*Name changed.

NOTE ON SOURCES

This book is a work of nonfiction, drawn upon primary materials from three principal sources: personal interviews with past and present employees of the American Red Cross, blood industry officials, regional blood bankers, research scientists, government officials, transfusion AIDS victims and their families and attorneys; court transcripts, depositions, FDA investigative reports, internal memos, letters, reports, charts, notes and meeting minutes from the American Red Cross and other blood industry organizations, suppliers and manufacturers and other pertinent documents that are part of the public record in the United States and Canada.

The names of some individuals, including the Wilson and Michaels families, have been changed to protect their privacy.

INTRODUCTION

BAD BLOOD began as an intellectual challenge in an information black-out. It became, over time, a parable.

In December 1995, I suggested to a leading women's magazine an article on "Extraordinary Women on the Campaign Trail." The Republican race had begun heating up and I decided to focus on Elizabeth Dole and her longtime protege, Mari Maseng-Will, wife of the conservative political essayist George Will. Mrs. Dole had recently taken a leave of absence from the Red Cross to devote herself to her husband's third bid for the presidency. Ms. Maseng-Will, a public relations powerhouse in Washington D.C., was Bob Dole's flamboyant speech writer and a key strategist. Two powerful women, two friends, a common cause.

I was told by the Dole campaign headquarters that any interviews with Mrs. Dole were arranged through the Red Cross. I called the Red Cross press department, asking for some background information on its president. A packet of articles arrived. Here was an inarguably accomplished woman who had served several presidents, but whose portfolio had been reduced to anecdotes about God and marriage, a religious awakening and late night "pillow talks" with her husband. I called again, this time with specific questions about Mrs. Dole's management style, the individuals on whom she relied for advice and potential conflicts with her husband's political aims. None of those questions were answered.

Instead, I received a call from the very agitated magazine editor-in-chief. She wanted to know "on whose authority" was I asking these questions? She told me to "cease and desist" and "get off this story," that she was "on the board of Mrs. Dole," whatever that meant. Subsequently I received another call, this one from the press officer at the Red Cross. He read a prepared statement to me: five times. That statement effectively dropped an iron curtain between me, the Red Cross and Elizabeth Dole. Mari Maseng-Will had already declined to be interviewed.

I did not know, then, just what it was I was looking for, only that I was told not to look. I had no idea what I would find, only that I wanted to know what had inspired such obstinance.

What I discovered was a profound sense of betrayal and fear. In the fifteen years I have been a member of the working press, covering a range of subjects from organized crime to scientific fraud, I have never encountered the kind of palpable anxiety expressed to me by numerous sources. Principal among their concerns were fears of reprisals from the Red Cross. As a result, many high-level officials currently and formerly associated with the organization spoke to me only on guarantee of anonymity.

I began receiving internal documents via mail and fax, the return address or phone number blackened out. As the months went by I felt as if I were involved in a covert operation, certainly not a story about the nation's most revered charity. As layers were peeled away, what became evident was a significant discrepancy between the Red Cross's public image and its operational policies. A benevolent persona versus an insular corporate culture.

Taking a critical look at this sacred American institution was a study in power, the power we so easily bestow through our blind trust. Regardless of their stated mission, institutions are not sacred. What is sacred is the truth.

CHAPTER ONE

THREE BABIES

I think Red Cross and the "powers that be" could have done something to avert these deaths. They just didn't have the guts to stand up.

Dr. Frank Saulsbury
University of Virginia

"Feel here, Mama, it's moving."

Jewelle Ann Michaels and her daughter-in-law, Debby, were sitting in Jewelle's kitchen, one of six tiny rooms in a cinderblock house in rural Southwest Virginia. The smell of spring—damp earth and daffodils pushing up toward the sunlight—drifted through the open window. It was, Jewelle thought, a time of renewal, the best time to be carrying a child. She laid her hand on Debby's taut, swollen belly and felt that familiar joyful kicking of new life. It would be her first grandchild, her son Jim's first baby.

The Michaels family had once been a prolific clan, descendants of patriot Patrick Henry and among the earliest settlers of the Blue Ridge Mountains. Craftsmen and carpenters, they had come from England and Scotland in the 1700s to build the capital city of Williamsburg and had stayed on to prosper. Nearly 300 years later, all that remained of their ancestral home, the glorious Plantation Gardens, were the cemetery's ancient gravemarkers and a few parcels of land with tinderbox houses scattered along a dirt road.

After a difficult first marriage, Jewelle had raised Jimmy on her own, in these small rooms. When he and Debby married and they learned she was pregnant, the couple moved into Jim's old bedroom and awaited the baby. They tried saving up enough to strike out on their own but still had trouble making ends meet. Jim had always wanted children. He was a good boy, a hard worker, born to be a family man. In less than five months, at age eighteen, he was going to be a father. Debby was seventeen.

Debby placed her own hand on the opposite side of her stomach. "It's moving here, too," she said.

Jewelle laughed when she felt yet more rapid kicking under her fingers. "Debby, honey," she said, "you got more than one baby in there. Because as small as this baby is, if it's moving here, you can't feel it moving way over there."

So Jewelle was not surprised when the doctor found two heartbeats. A few weeks later, ultrasound picked up the third.

When they drove to Jim's job at a local factory and told him in the parking lot that Debby was going to have three babies, not two, he turned pale and collapsed up against a parked car. "Oh, my God, she's joking, right?"

They all hugged and cried, and then Debby and Jim asked her how they'd all manage.

"We'll just buy three of everything," Jewelle said.

Debby was nearly seven months pregnant when she experienced terrible pains in her stomach. Jim checked her into Virginia Baptist Hospital, but when the doctors there learned she was expecting triplets, they transferred her to the University of Virginia. It had the facilities for handling multiple, and what looked like premature, births. On July 2, 1984, Debby gave birth to three identical girls. Each weighed about two pounds. Jim was not allowed into the delivery room.

He was standing with his mother in the hallway when the nurse wheeled the infants past him. They were lying in an incubator, and they were very tiny.

The doctor told Jim that the third baby almost didn't make it. All three had needed a small amount of blood, which was not unusual for such premature births. The third baby remained in intensive care for two more weeks because of respiratory problems. She needed several blood transfusions.

The infants were subsequently transferred to Virginia Baptist Hospital, where they would remain for at least two more months, time enough to develop to term.

Jim left their naming up to Debby. For a while, they were babies A, B, and C. Jewelle knit three tiny hats, each embroidered with a yellow letter. Hats that could have only fit three small "doll babies,"

Jewelle told Debby as they tied them under the girls' tiny chins, dressed them in doll clothes, and brought them home.

By then they had been named in the order in which they were born: Heather, Holly, Hailey.

It was hard to tell them apart, but their personalities soon emerged. Holly was the leader of the three. Hailey was a clown who loved to entertain with funny faces. Heather was quieter, the more delicate.

There was never any sibling rivalry. If anything, the girls seemed astonishingly attuned to each other. They had an intuitive sense of what each felt and wanted. Sometimes Jewelle wondered whether the girls were just one person whose soul had been divided into three.

They had the usual childhood diseases—colds, and problems with ears, noses, and throats. No sooner would one girl get well than the next would fall ill. Their infections seemed to last a long time and never fully disappear. Nonetheless they were happy, rarely cried, and never complained. They loved music, loved to dance and dress up. They often laughed and grinned at the same time.

The Michaelses' world revolved around the triplets. Jim worked double shifts to earn more money, and Debby took on a part-time job. Jewelle scheduled her own shifts at a cookie factory so that she could be with the girls. Somehow, they all managed in Jewelle's cramped quarters.

One morning in early March 1985, eight-month-old Hailey awoke covered with tiny purplish spots. It was, Jewelle observed, as if someone had taken a pen and dotted her entire body. She called the girls' pediatrician. Did he know what was wrong with Hailey? She'd never seen anything like it.

Dr. Frank Saulsbury, a pediatric immunologist at the University of Virginia, had not chosen medicine in order to attend funerals of children. But death came with the territory. Saulsbury's specialty was treating kids with immunodeficiencies and auto-immune disorders like lupus. He also saw what was commonly dubbed "bubble babies," children whose defenses against infection were so poor that minor infections resisted by healthy individuals could prove devastating, if not fatal.

Saulsbury was attending physician on the general inpatient ward service and occasionally consulted at NICU, the neonatal intensive care unit. One morning in August 1983, he was discussing some cases with a young resident, Dr. Randy Wykoff. When they reviewed the young patients' charts they were struck by the condition of three of the children. A boy and two girls, each eight months old, were suffering unusual illnesses, which raised questions about their immune functioning.

Wykoff recognized these children from their last hospitalization at NICU in November 1982. Here they were back again at the same time, less than one year later.

It was, Saulsbury remarked, a strange coincidence.

Saulsbury was aware from his readings of an emerging immunodeficiency disease called AIDS. By August 1983, compelling evidence suggested transfusion-associated AIDS in adults and children. There had been at least one documented case of transfusion AIDS in San Francisco. A baby had received about twenty blood transfusions and subsequently died of AIDS. One of the blood donors in that case was a gay man who later died of AIDS.

While he conducted diagnostic tests on the three infants, Saulsbury reviewed their NICU records. He found what he was looking for: all had been transfused at birth with packed red blood cells. He then checked the blood unit number. Each child had received blood from the same single unit, which had been split three ways. It was a common practice to divide up a unit of blood among premature infants since only small quantities were required. That unit had been obtained from a single donor. Saulsbury also learned that another infant who had been in NICU had received blood from that unit. That child's whereabouts were unknown.

The University of Virginia obtained blood from the American Red Cross for its 650-bed facility. The blood came from Red Cross's Washington, D.C. center, which was over 100 miles away. UVA Medical Center contacted the Red Cross which cooperated in locating the donor.

The donor was found in November.

His blood was tested at the National Institutes of Health laboratory of Dr. Robert Gallo. Gallo had been working on several assays which could detect the presence of antibodies to a virus called HTLV-III, which was under investigation as the cause of AIDS, (it would later be confirmed as the cause and renamed "HIV" for the Human Immunodeficiency Virus). The presence of serum antibody to HTLV-III was believed to be diagnostic of AIDS or to indicate a serious risk of the disease. Antibody to the virus was virtually never present in the serum of healthy adults who were not members of AIDS risk groups. Although there was no comparable data concerning HTLV-III antibody in healthy children, there was no reason to suspect that the antibody status of normal children was different than that of normal healthy adults. Saulsbury sent samples of the infants' blood to Gallo.

The children's test results came back: each was infected with HTLV-III. So was the donor.

The mothers of the infants were not tested for HTLV-III antibody, but maternal transmission was exceedingly unlikely, since none of the mothers were members of an AIDS high-risk group. Nor did they have sexual partners at risk for AIDS. Saulsbury concluded that his young patients had contracted HTLV-III infection through transfusion of blood from a common donor who was asymptomatically infected.

The University of Virginia physician had recorded the first, documented cases of transfusion AIDS caused by a single unit of blood traced back to one donor. He informed the Red Cross's D.C. center of his findings. As Saulsbury would later recall by February 1984, "Red Cross knew damn good and well they had a problem here."

Saulsbury would later identify these three transfusion AIDS babies as Cohort A.

In late February 1985, three more children with similar immune disorders were admitted to the University of Virginia Medical Center. One boy seemed to have a congenital immunodeficiency disease, except that his identical twin brother was healthy. Another baby had thrombocytopenia, a drastic reduction in the number of blood platelets that resulted in abnormal bleeding: this in turn, caused purpura, small purplish dots on the skin. Thrombocytopenia may be due to an auto-immune disorder, or follow a viral infection. It was unusual to see it in an infant. The third showed similar immune deficiencies. All three had been in NICU during September 1983. All had received blood at birth from a common unit of blood from one donor. When Saulsbury had these children's blood tested with the commercially available AIDS test, the results came back positive for HIV antibodies. The boy's twin had also received multiple blood transfusions at birth, but from a different, noninfected donor; he tested negative. By the time Saulsbury received the blood test results, the little girl had died; she was nine months old.

He identified this second set of three HIV babies as Cohort B. The donor to Cohort B would test positive for HIV in March 1986, when he returned to donate blood for the third time at the Red Cross. But in the interim his second donation had already been processed and transfused.

Subsequently, Saulsbury became intrigued by a case described to him by a friend and colleague, Dr. Tom Howard. Howard, a hematologist, told him about an eight-month-old patient he had seen in March. She had developed thrombocytopenia. After a course of treatment, the baby had recovered and showed no further symptoms. Saulsbury did not yet know that he would be looking at the first member of Cohort C, who had received blood from the same donor as Cohort B. Saulsbury suggested that the Michaels bring in their daughter Hailey, and her two sisters right away.

All three girls had contracted transfusion AIDS.

By the end of 1985, a dozen children suffering transfusion-AIDS had been seen at the University of Virginia Medical Center. Nine of those cases—the triplets among them—had been caused by a single donor who had given blood several times at the American Red Cross's Washington, D.C. center.

Neither Jim nor Debby knew much about AIDS. Jim told Saulsbury he thought AIDS came from homosexuals. What did blood have to do with it? Were the girls going to get better? Wasn't there anything he could do?

Saulsbury explained to Jim that he had nothing to offer. There was no cure; their prognosis was fatal. At best, he could only modify the time and mode of the girls' deaths to make it as bearable as possible.

When Jim told his mother, Jewelle said they would surely find a cure.

The first time Frank Saulsbury pulled into the Michaels's driveway, it was a bleak, cold day. A light rain fell on the girls' swing set.

The cinderblock house was very modest. The spare surroundings contrasted sharply with his impression of his young patients, who were always dressed "to the nines, like young preppies." The triplets were extraordinarily bright and upbeat—precocious, really.

Saulsbury had already met their grandmother and knew she was the source of the girls' extraordinary vitality. Jewelle Ann Michaels was an amazing woman. What she lacked in financial resources she more than compensated for in love and absolute devotion. It was clear that she had led a difficult life, made no easier by the sickness of her granddaughters, but she had not become bitter. She was the backbone of strength and optimism in the family. And she had clearly decided that whatever time they had on this earth would be happy. The girls idolized her.

For the first few years, apart from protracted childhood illnesses, the girls led normal lives. Their favorite foods were "Granny's smashed potatoes," "bizdits [biscuits] and gravy," and pizza. They adored ice cream and preferred cake to pie or pudding. They always watched *Little House on the Prairie*. Holly's favorite color was blue, Heather's purple, Hailey's pink. They would hear a song once and be able to sing it word for word. Every night after their bath they would dress up in pink tutus and Jewelle would put their hair up "like big girls." Then they tap-danced and sang. Heather, who liked playing drums, was the most musical.

All three girls loved to ride in the car with Jewelle when it rained. "Turn your wind-shippers on, Granny," Holly would say. "It's rinkin'."

When they were two, they watched their dog, Baby, give birth to a litter of five puppies. They sat beside Baby in their little sundresses and Holly exclaimed, "Oh gosh, Granny, another one is popping out!" They were convinced that their great-grandma, Jewelle's mother Nona, who lived next door, was going to have puppies because her stomach was as big as Baby's had been.

When they were three, they drove their Barbie cars as if they had been driving for years. They backed out of the driveway and tore off down the dirt road like teenagers as Jim ran alongside them.

When Hailey was three, she again developed thrombocytopenia, a common feature of HIV in adults and children. Saulsbury's article for the *Journal of Pediatrics* in 1986, based on his observations of Hailey and HIV infants, recommended that physicians consider a diagnosis of HTLV-III infection infants with thrombocytopenia. This time, though, Hailey did not fully respond to prednisone (a corticosteroid to reduce inflammation and treat blood disorders). Her platelet count remained low. With a diminished immune system, Hailey was prone to continual infection.

Heather and Holly were four years old when they first showed symptoms of AIDS. Heather developed swollen lymph nodes. Holly developed severe thrombocytopenia. There was barely an inch of her body not covered with purplish sores. Like Heather, Holly did not respond to prednisone or to intravenous immunoglobin, made from blood serum and containing antibodies that fight disease. As her condition persisted, her spleen became enlarged. In July 1989, when she was five, Holly had her spleen removed. Her platelet count promptly increased and her condition improved.

By the end of that year all three were on AZT. A new antiviral drug, AZT inhibited the replication of HIV. By slowing down the spread of the virus, the drug helped relieve symptoms. It had proved beneficial to adults and was particularly helpful in reversing thrombocytopenia.

Yet even when they were ill, the girls thought of others. "Don't worry, Granny," they told Jewelle, when they saw her look away with tears in her eyes. "Be happy."

By the time his children began showing symptoms, Jim Michaels had read just about everything he could find about AIDS. He conveyed this information to Debby and his mother. Jewelle learned about white and red blood cells, platelets, T-cell counts, lesions. So when the girls developed what looked like chicken pox and she and Jim would sit up with them for hours, gently patting their raw skin with a tissue, she knew enough to ask Saulsbury: was this really chicken pox, or could it be shingles or herpes? But when the girls said, "It hurts so bad, Granny," it didn't much matter to Jewelle what name the doctor gave the sores and lesions.

As their bouts with illness became more frequent, Jewelle Michaels watched her son Jim struggle to contain his rage. "I just don't see how this happened to my girls," he kept saying. "Someone messed up real bad."

CHAPTER TWO

MAGIC MAN

If you are well, then you probably have not been exposed.

Letter to Roland Ray
from Suburban Hospital,
Bethesda, Maryland

Roland Ray had just rung up what he thought was his last sale of the day when two young black men walked into his convenience store, the Corner Beer and Wine, and asked if he carried California Wine Coolers. They were about nineteen or twenty years old. One wore a bright yellow fishnet tank top and jeans; the other, ripped jeans. Roland told them the cold wine was in the refrigerator by the back wall. He then returned to tallying the week's receipts.

It was nearly midnight, but on sweltering nights like this one in mid-August, it was not uncommon for residents near Diamond Avenue in the Maryland community of Gaithersburg to pick up a cool drink or a pack of cigarettes right before closing time. Roland never worried about staying open so late. At 6´4˝ and 250 pounds, with a bushy blond beard, he was an imposing figure.

But to those who knew him, Roland Ray was a gentle giant.

Roland had come by way of carpentry and home appliance sales to set up, with his father's help, his own business. He and his dad had always been close—hiking, fishing, swapping handy work at each other's houses, amicably competing over who grew the biggest tomatoes. Their business partnership worked. Roland was well liked by the communities he served, but the store's selling wine and beer had created friction between the dry, affluent enclave of Washington Grove and the nearby low-income housing development. The Washington Grovers resented their largely black neighbors traipsing through their oak-shaded streets on the way to Roland's store. The feud had heated up, along with the temperature. It was not simply for economic reasons that Roland had stood his ground. Many of those poorer families were as hardworking as his own, struggling to make ends meet and keep their children off the streets. Roland had become a role model for many of those kids, a big white guy in his early thirties who did magic tricks and encouraged them to stay in school.

They had named him "Magic Man."

Roland saw the men approach the counter with a four-pack. The one in the yellow shirt asked for E-Z Wide rolling papers. It was shelved alongside the cigarettes, behind the counter. Roland turned back to the register and looked straight at the muzzle of a chrome-plated .44. It was so close he could see a silver bullet in its big barrel.

From the corner of his eye he saw the second man aiming a handgun at his chest. They wanted the money. To open the cash drawer, Roland had to punch in a few more keys. The man in yellow panicked. "He's hitting the alarm!" he shouted.

Roland said, "I don't have—"

Then he heard the shot. The impact spun him around and flung him on top of the cooler of soda he kept behind the counter. He didn't feel any pain, just shock. The guy in ripped jeans started pounding the register's keys.

Roland told him to break it open. They took all the cash, about $700, and ran.

The pain was gathering in his chest, like a beesting that intensified and fanned out. Roland yanked the phone to the floor and dialed 911. He told the dispatcher his store had been robbed, he'd been shot in the stomach, and he needed an ambulance. Was he bleeding? Roland touched his stomach and felt the warm fluid. Yes, he was.

Roland lay the receiver on the floor beside his head and waited. He heard the dispatcher tell him to "hang in there." The burning sensation ripped through his limbs. He wondered whether he was going to die or be paralyzed. He closed his eyes and thought about his kids, Sandra and Wayne. That day, August 14, 1984, was Wayne's sixth birthday.

The store was suddenly packed with police officers and paramedics. Two men rolled him onto the stretcher. They were telling him he was going to be okay. He asked one of them to call his father, not his wife; he knew she would get scared. He kept thinking about Sandra and Wayne, and what would happen if he died.

Roland made all kinds of bargains with God as they wheeled him into the night. Darkness shivered around the whirring yellow ambulance light. He felt the crowd that had gathered press in around him. Someone shouted, "Hey, Magic Man!" Someone, maybe one of the paramedics, said something about his losing a lot of blood. They hooked him up to an IV unit and the ambulance screeched out onto Route 270.

The hospital at Shady Grove was closest, but they told him they were taking him to Suburban Hospital in Bethesda. It had a trauma unit.

Then he passed out.

Roland drifted in and out of consciousness as the stretcher slid out of the van and a flurry of white coats descended upon him. He was wheeled into the operating room. Someone was cutting off his damp clothes. He heard a woman's soft voice say, "Roland, you're going into surgery. You are going to be okay."

Dr. Daniel Powers, chief surgeon at Suburban's trauma ward, happened to be on call that night. Powers worked quickly in the OR. Roland's right lung had not collapsed, but there was a large bullet wound in the dome of his liver. Powers brought forward the entire liver so that he could fully examine it. It was raw and oozing, bleeding profusely. Roland's stomach was severely distended and filled with blood. Powers controlled the bleeding with figure-eight sutures and packing, and he ordered two units of blood transfused.

There was no evidence the bullet had exited Roland's body. An X ray showed it was still lodged below his diaphragm, to the right of his spine. Powers could not remove the bullet without risking damage to Roland's spinal cord. He decided to wait until it migrated into a safer zone, most likely the tissue of Roland's back, below the skin, a process that would take about two weeks.

Roland was running a high fever. He was lucid one moment and drifted off into a dreamlike state the next. When he regained consciousness, his first request was for a phone: he had to speak to his kids. They were crying, scared, as he expected. "Dad, we love you," they told him. Roland said he was going to come home soon.

He began to improve slowly and was transferred to the ICU. There his family kept watch. Hooked up to tubes, he felt utterly and un-characteristically helpless. But when he heard the reassuring voices of his parents, his four sisters and brother, and his uncles and aunts, he felt well loved.

Six weeks into his recovery, the store was again robbed. Sandra and Wayne had been there only hours earlier with their mother. Roland decided it was time to close up and move on. He began driving a cab. Then, when his strength returned, he worked construction jobs with his brother-in-law. His marriage ended, but he had been awarded custody of Wayne, and soon Sandra decided to live with him as well. In 1987, Roland fell in love with a soft-spoken young woman. Janet worked at a daycare center and was studying elementary education in college. They shared the same goals: to have a big family and a comfortable house with a yard, and to live what Roland called the "American dream."

Their first child, Emily, was born in February 1989.

A few months later, on the morning of June 15, Roland Ray was at a jobsite in Washington, D.C. when the foreman called him to the office. Janet was on the phone. Roland was supposed to pick up Wayne after school, and he figured the plans had changed. His wife's voice sounded odd. She told him he had received a letter from Suburban Hospital, and that he'd better sit down. He asked her to read it to him. The letter was from Dr. Robert Chambers, chairman of the Department of Pathology.

Dear Mr. Roland, [sic]

We here at Suburban Hospital Blood Bank have recently been informed by our blood supplier, the American Red Cross, that a blood donor who donated blood used by you during your surgical admission for a gunshot wound in 1984, on return for further donation, is positive for the virus associated with Acquired Immune Deficiency Syndrome, AIDS.

No testing for the AIDS virus was available in 1984, so there was no way then to know whether the donor was infected. There is a good possibility that the donor was not infected at the time of the donation in 1984; however, we cannot be sure and recommend that you return to the Suburban Hospital laboratory for testing. I should point out that if you are well, then you probably have not been exposed as a result of that blood transfusion. But nevertheless, for protection of those near to you and your own peace of mind, please return for testing. There will be no charge to you.

At first they thought it was some kind of sick joke. It had been five years since the robbery and his surgery. Why had the hospital taken so long to contact him?

What neither Roland nor Janet knew then was that Red Cross had learned on May 9, 1985—four years earlier—that Roland Ray's blood donor had tested HIV positive. Red Cross had taken four years to inform the hospital.

They told each other there was probably nothing to worry about. *If you are well, then you probably have not been exposed . . .* He was well.

When he and Janet returned to Suburban, they spent five minutes in Dr. Chambers's office. There was time enough for Chambers to draw blood, but the doctor had no time for their rapid-fire questions. How did this happen? they wanted to know. They had a four-month-old baby. Could she be sick? What about Janet?

"We'll call you," Dr. Chambers said, as they were ushered out the door.

Roland and his wife waited all weekend to hear the blood test results. He and Janet sat at the dining room table while the children slept, and they went around and around in circles, like sleepwalkers. They had married for love, they were still in love. They cried a lot.

On Sunday, Roland and Janet went to his parents' house, a mile from theirs. The Rays were having a family get-together—no special occasion, just an excuse for everyone to visit. Roland had decided to tell his family about the letter from Suburban and the blood test. They had always been close. In times of need, whether emotional or financial, the family banded together for comfort and support. Now he needed them, and their prayers. Roland told his siblings and his parents he had to talk to them in private. They all went into his parents' bedroom.

No one knew what to say. His mothers and sisters cried. Roland told his dad how afraid he was about Janet and Emily. He could not live with himself if he had infected them.

In late October, Mike Feldman, a partner with the D.C. law firm Ashcraft & Gerel, received a phone call from Bob Samet, a partner in the firm's Rockville, Maryland office. Samet relayed to Feldman a recent conversation he'd had with a client for whom he had obtained some workman's compensation in 1985. The client, a man named Roland Ray, had been shot during a robbery of his convenience store in the summer of 1984. Ray had had a blood transfusion during surgery. In August 1989, he had learned that he had contracted AIDS from the transfusion. The blood had come from the Red Cross. Feldman told Samet to refer Roland to him.

For the past two years, Mike Feldman and his colleagues had been thrashing through largely uncharted, hostile territory: they had been battling the Red Cross, an American icon.

It began for Feldman in the spring of 1987, when a middle-aged black woman named Rita Wilson walked into the D.C. offices of Ashcraft & Gerel. She had been referred by the firm's Virginia office. Mrs. Wilson sat across from Feldman and, wiping away tears, began telling him about her daughter, Andrea. Andrea was born on October 2, 1974. When she was six months old, she was diagnosed with sickle cell anemia, an inherited blood disorder, which caused chronic severe anemia and impeded blood flow. As a result of this illness, in late November 1981 Andrea suffered a "cerebral vascular accident." The stroke affected the right side of her brain. In September 1982, Andrea suffered a second stroke, again affecting the right side of her brain. She found it difficult to use her left hand. On October 1, she entered the Children's Hospital National Medical Center. The physicians there scheduled her to receive blood transfusions on a routine basis in order to avoid another stroke.

In mid-July 1984, Andrea returned for her regular monthly blood transfusion. Unknown to her, the transfusion she received had been contaminated with HIV. The blood had been provided to the hospital by the American Red Cross.

Children's Hospital told Mrs. Wilson that, although there was a chance Andrea would get AIDS, it was more likely she would not, that she would be fine.

Andrea had, indeed, been infected. The HIV damaged her already weak immune system. She became susceptible to various illnesses. She could not eat because of the herpes sores in her mouth. She could not go to school or play with her friends. She developed pneumonia. Her liver became swollen. Her skin darkened dramatically.

On May 16, 1987, after years of suffering, Andrea was hospitalized for pneumonia, she fell into a coma and never regained consciousness. On June 18, 1987, she died. She was thirteen years old.

Long and lean, with silvery dark hair, Mike Feldman was quick to assess people and situations, and when he took on a case, it became his cause. The part of him that had rejected corporate law, that loved the challenge of "going after the big bad guys who wronged the little guys," drew him to the plaintiff firm. He had taken on Agent Orange and asbestos cases, filed suit against the Washington Metro Transit Authority, and brought some of the major D.C. hospitals to court. His clients were ordinary people to whom extraordinarily unfair things had happened.

Feldman's track record was impressive, and few situations surprised him. But what Rita Wilson was telling him stunned him. Feldman knew little about AIDS, even less about transfusion AIDS, except what he had heard on television news reports and read in the popular press. But he knew a lot more about the Red Cross . . . who didn't? For over a hundred years, the American Red Cross had cultivated and, as far as Feldman knew, earned the public's trust. It had become to America's collective unconscious as emblematic as the American flag. Feldman did not know whether Mrs. Wilson had a negligence case, and if so, against whom, the hospital or the Red Cross. If the Red Cross were implicated, he would be taking on much more than a damages award case. He would be battling an institution built on decades of goodwill.

Which was just how his associate, Chris Tisi, reacted when Feldman strode into his office to discuss the case.

Christopher Tisi was in his late twenties, virtually fresh out of law school, boyish. He had an ingenuous quality which set him apart from the stereotypical portrait of a lawyer. People liked Tisi; they trusted him. Civic minded, Tisi had often organized Red Cross bloodmobile drives while in college.

He told Feldman, "Are you nuts? Suing the Red Cross would be like going after Mother Teresa."

Still, they shopped the idea around the office, among the twenty or so attorneys and clerical staff. Over and over again they heard the same refrain: "Go after the Red Cross? Isn't *anything* sacred?"

At the end of that day, Feldman and Tisi had come to the same conclusion: "Yes," they replied. "The truth."

By the time Roland Ray met Mike Feldman and Chris Tisi in the fall of 1989, the lawyers had already filed the Wilson lawsuit. They had lost their naïveté, but not their sense of moral outrage. When, in 1987, they charged the Red Cross with negligence in causing the death of Andrea Wilson, they expected a battle. They did not expect war. The Red Cross displayed the kind of legal aggression which often characterized lawsuits involving Fortune 500 corporations.

The fact that Red Cross blood collected prior to 1985 had been tainted with a fatal, contagious disease transmissible by IV drug users and homosexual men did not reflect well on an organization whose most bankable asset was its good name. In addition to the 4 million people each year who donated blood, a cadre of 1.4 million volunteers, and tens of millions of dollars in free television, radio, and print ads—one-third of which went to promoting its blood program—the Red Cross boasted a nationwide network of 52 regional blood centers, an impressive Washington, D.C. headquarters dubbed the "Marble Palace," 2,817 chapters, a multimillion-dollar research lab, and a closed-circuit TV network and a production studio. Its vast reservoir of goodwill enabled it to procure, for free, millions of units of blood, which it converted into a half-billion-dollar commodity in fiscal 1988. That amount represented 53 percent of its $985 million in revenues. Red Cross's net worth was then nearly $1 billion, and its cash and investments were worth nearly $560 million. It was also a major player in the commercial plasma business, claiming about a 15 percent share of the U.S. market; its sales of plasma that year alone amounted to a tax-free $75 million.

Had the Red Cross been a "for profit" business, its total revenues would have placed it number 339 on the 1988 Fortune 500 list. Its enviable 8.7 percent profit margin would have ranked it ahead of GE and Mobil Oil.

It also contracted with the powerful D.C. law firm Arnold & Porter, to which it paid millions of dollars to fight claims of liability brought by transfusion AIDS victims.

Arnold & Porter, whose clients included tobacco giant Philip Morris, coordinated the Red Cross's national litigation strategy. The Red Cross could not afford a loss here, or a loss there, any errant precedents that could open a window of opportunity for transfusion AIDS victims to sue successfully.

There was no room for error. There could be no leaks in the dam.

As the Ashcraft & Gerel attorneys would discover, the Red Cross strategy seemed to be "divide, conquer, and bury."

Central to Red Cross's successful defense was public ignorance. To that end it was important that any internal policy documents be kept strictly confidential. It could not risk the kind of exposure involved in discovery motions, in which opposing counsel requested production of documents. Many of these documents reflected the evolution in the Red Cross's thinking about AIDS, the internal deliberative processes by which it opted in 1983 not to test blood or directly question donors who were at high-risk for AIDS. Some of these documents appeared to indicate organizational priorities which placed image and money above public safety. Consequently, Red Cross routinely requested that the courts put under "protective order" litigation documents. It argued that disclosure of sensitive internal communications would create undue public anxiety over events which had occurred in the past. Such doubts could, the Red Cross claimed, result in decreased donations and endanger the adequacy of the blood supply.

Overloaded courts were more than willing to accede to the Red Cross's requests. Judges more often than not opted for expediency over the public interest and granted carte blanche protective orders. Thus the public and media were denied access to thousands of sensitive Red Cross documents.

In effect, a legal "bubble" had been created around the Red Cross. Each victim's lawsuit had to be constructed from ground zero, in contrast to the Red Cross's centralized, cohesive defense.

Ironically, the Red Cross had been founded a hundred years earlier to protect and assist the kinds of victims it now so aggressively fought . . . people who had become victims of the Red Cross itself.

CHAPTER THREE

ANGEL OF MERCY
1861–1981

*There is no doubt that the day is not far distant—if it has
not already come—when the American people will
recognize the Red Cross as one of the wisest and best
systems of philanthropic work in modern times.*

Daily Journal, Evanston, Illinois
April 3, 1884

Clara Barton was part of a generation of women at the end of the
Victorian Age who found dwindling opportunity to marry and, instead, took up careers as ministers, teachers, or social workers. Barton was in her forties before she found her calling.

What aroused in her the undaunted passion to tend to the
sick and wounded is a matter of historical question. But nothing
apparent in the personal history of this diminutive, school-
teacher–turned–government clerk portended her groundbreaking
role in public health. When the Civil War erupted and President
Abraham Lincoln issued a call for volunteers in April 1861, Clara
Barton answered. Leveraging her political connections, Barton solicited volunteers and contributions of supplies to aid the Union soldiers in her home state of Massachusetts. When the first wounded
arrived bloodied and bandaged in Washington, D.C., Barton was
there, along with a number of Washington women she had recruited.

For more than a year, Barton served the Union from the nation's
capital. But the battlefields called her. U.S. policy barred women
from the front, so she launched a one-woman crusade. Her lobbying efforts paid off. On August 12, 1862, she was permitted to go to
war. In her diary, she wrote that she removed the hoop from her
skirt, donned a plaid jacket and dark skirt, loaded her supplies, and

drove a four-mule team alone to the Battle of Culpepper. From that time on, wherever the battle raged, Barton was there, with nursing assistance, hot soup, and fresh-baked bread, earning her the reputation as an "Angel of Mercy." She was undaunted by the carnage. "I wrung the blood from the bottom of my clothing before I could step from the weight about my feet," she wrote of her experience at the front. Her heroic ministerings to soldiers were the subject of daily newspaper dispatches, and her reputation grew among the rain-soaked, battle-weary soldiers of the Union. One, a brigade surgeon, wrote of Barton, "I thought that night if heaven ever sent out a holy angel she must be one, her assistance was so timely."

Barton was present at the final battles of the Civil War in 1865 and during the process of identifying the dead. At President Lincoln's authority she created the Bureau of Missing Persons, which after four arduous years, identified 20,000 dead who would otherwise have remained anonymous. After the war, Barton traveled to Europe to recuperate. It was there that she learned of the International Red Cross movement.

The movement had begun in the mid-nineteenth century, when a Swiss banker, Jean Henri Dumont, on holiday in Italy, had stumbled upon the aftermath of a battle fought between the Austrian Army and a coalition of French and Sardinians. Near the village of Solferino, he discovered 30,000 to 40,000 men; some dead, many dying. Dumont rallied doctors and volunteers from the surrounding villages to tend to the wounded. Subsequently, he returned to Switzerland, but the experience left its mark. In 1862 Dumont wrote *Un Souvenir de Solferino,* which issued a call to "press forward in a humane and truly civilized spirit the attempt to prevent, or at least to alleviate, the horrors of war." Dumont's work was dubbed by a French historian "the greatest work of the century."

In response, a group of Swiss scholars organized the movement that became the International Committee of Red Cross, and was officially sanctioned at the Geneva Convention on August 22, 1864. Its motif: the reverse of the Swiss flag, which was a white cross on a red background. By 1866, twenty-two nations had signed the Treaty of Geneva, which provided neutrality for hospitals and ambulances and the care of all wounded soldiers regardless of nationality. The Red Cross emblem was adopted as a symbol of neutrality. Isolationism and fear of international entanglements kept the United States from joining. Outraged, Barton wrote in her diary, "Not a civilized people in the world but ourselves is missing. I began to fear that in the eyes of the rest of mankind we could not be far from barbarianism."

Barton remained in Europe for four years, working with the International Red Cross relief efforts during the Franco-Prussian War. When she returned to the States, she began a five-year lobbying effort for U.S. approval of the Geneva Convention. Finally she could wait no longer. On May 21, 1881, Barton called together a small group of friends and associates in Washington, D.C. to organize "the greatest venture of voluntary service in the world": the American Association of the Red Cross. In addition to its performing wartime relief services, Barton envisioned the Red Cross in a peacetime role, providing assistance to victims of natural disaster.

On July 26, 1882, the United States signed the Treaty of Geneva and the American Red Cross received official recognition. Barton was sixty-one at the time.

From June 8, 1881 to May 14, 1904, Clara Barton served as president of the American Red Cross. Under her leadership, Red Cross volunteers provided relief to the victims of twenty-one natural disasters, including fires, floods, and hurricanes, as well as to Russian peasants in the famine of 1892 and to Armenian victims of Turkish persecution in 1896. Just as she had driven mule carts to Civil War battlefields thirty-six years earlier, she did the same during the Spanish American War at age seventy-four. One of her co-workers, Judge Joseph Seldon, praised Barton at the International Red Cross convention in 1884: "She has done her work with the skill of a statesman, the heart of a woman, and the final perseverance of the saints."

While Barton's hands-on style made her beloved among the American people, her prolonged absences from Red Cross headquarters drew criticism from within the organization. A faction of the Red Cross Executive Committee, members led by longtime volunteer Mabel Boardman, charged that Barton's inability to delegate responsibility and her lack of attention to accounting and management were harming the organization. A woman of privileged background, Boardman had powerful political connections. She was able to orchestrate a congressional investigation of the Red Cross. But no evidence was found to implicate Barton in anything more than sloppy accounting. The investigation was terminated by Senator Redfield Proctor, who characterized it as "the most outrageous proceeding that has ever come under observation." Her reputation intact, Barton resigned from the Red Cross in 1904. The

Chicago Inter-Ocean wrote, "Clara Barton cannot resign her place in the world as the one real true representative of the Red Cross in this country."

Indeed, she had not resigned from her philanthropic mission.

At the age of eighty-two, Barton formed the National First Aid Association of America, which worked in tandem with the Red Cross until her death on April 12, 1912, at the age of ninety.

Mabel Boardman never officially chaired the organization ("The chairman should always be a man," she wrote), but she ruled the Red Cross from behind the scenes for the next four decades. Hers was an organization dominated by individuals of social standing and prestige.

The American Red Cross was officially reorganized in a bill signed by President Roosevelt on January 5, 1905. Its purpose:

> *To furnish volunteer aid to the sick and wounded of armies in times of war . . .*
>
> *To perform all the duties devolved upon a national society by each nation which has acceded to [the Treaty of Geneva] . . .*
>
> *To act in matters of voluntary relief and in accord with the military and naval authorities as a medium of communication between the people of the United States of America and their Army and Navy . . .*
>
> *To continue and carry on a system of national and international relief in time of peace and apply the same in mitigating the sufferings caused by pestilence, famine, fire, floods, and other great national calamities, and to devise and carry on measures for preventing the same.*

The charter established a governing body, the Central Committee, which had direct government representation. Of its eighteen members, six were elected by the incorporators, six were elected by state or territorial societies, and six were appointed by the President of the United States. Five of those presidential nominees included the heads of the Departments of State, War, Navy, the Treasury, and Justice. The Red Cross was required to submit an annual auditing to the War Department for presentation to Congress.

Between 1905 and U.S. entry into World War I, Red Cross established prevention-oriented services and safety programs that remained a staple of its peacetime activities. Fundraising became a priority. Dances, bazaars, creative fundraisers like "Kick the Kaiser," and corporate gift-giving from the likes of American Tobacco swelled the Red Cross treasury from $200,000 in 1914 to $40 million in 1916.

As political tensions in Europe made the prospect of war inevitable, the tenor of the Red Cross adapted to a crisis orientation. On August 22, 1911, President William Howard Taft appointed the Red Cross, by charter, as "the only volunteer society now authorized by this government to render aid to its land and naval forces in war." When in 1914 Europe was plunged into war, the American Red Cross mobilized, dispatching its "Mercy Ship" to foreign ports in need.

By 1917, the Red Cross moved into its spectacular Washington, D.C. headquarters. It had already recruited 8,000 nurses, trained and ready for deployment to military hospitals; they quickly became America's sweethearts. President Woodrow Wilson established the charity as "an efficient arm of the government." Its newly created War Council was headed by J. P. Morgan and financier Henry P. Davison. By 1918, Red Cross membership topped an astounding 20 million and its payroll hovered at 14,000.

Following World War I, when Red Cross focused its efforts on America, humorist Will Rogers wrote, "We are so used to the things the Red Cross does that we sometimes just forget to praise them. Lord, what a blessing an organization like that is. I would have rather originated the Red Cross than to have written the Constitution of the United States."

In 1934, the Federal Emergency Relief Agency was established with $500 million appropriated by Congress for work and home relief programs. A product of President Franklin Delano Roosevelt's New Deal, FERA assumed many programs managed by the Red Cross. But as the Depression drew to a close, the Red Cross found its niche in national disaster relief mission.

But it was World War II that provided the charity with a heightened sense of purpose and the seeds of a lucrative business. In September 1939, when Germany invaded Poland, and Great Britain and France joined the war, American neutrality gave way to a fervor for defending democracy. On May 10, 1940, when Germany invaded Belgium and Holland, the Red Cross chairman, Norman Davis, former Undersecretary of State, launched a $20 million fundraising drive for European aid; the goal was swiftly met.

When the Japanese attacked Pearl Harbor, the Red Cross stepped up its efforts. Billboards, posters, placards, and radio, newspaper, and magazine ads emblazoned the slogan "Keep Your Red Cross at His Side." Dozens of magazine covers depicted Red Cross's ministries. The film *Seeing Him Through*, produced by Red Cross, was shown in 15,000 movie theaters. Millions of Americans were mobilized as volunteers. Scores of Red Cross workers earned military decoration, including three Silver Stars for gallantry in action. Over $700 million was raised, bankrolling Red Cross relief efforts into every military installation in the U.S. Its overseas aid extended into the European theater and to the far reaches of the Middle East, Africa, the Pacific, Australia, and Japan.

But it was the Red Cross's war-driven blood service that propelled the organization into the monied ranks of its corporate sponsors.

The first recorded transfusion appeared to have been performed on June 15, 1667 by French scientist Jean Baptiste Denis. Denis transfused the blood of a lamb into a fifteen-year-old boy, effectively marking the first animal-to-human organ transplant. But the practice was short lived. When another recipient of lamb's blood died, the surgeon was tried for murder. He was acquitted, but transfusions were abandoned for the next two centuries.

In the 1800s, new weapons of war inflicted wounds causing massive blood losses, and interest in transfusion was revived. Still, the procedure remained almost as risky as getting shot. Blood was transfused via a rubber syringe from the vein of the donor to the recipient. One in four patients suffered violent, sometimes fatal, allergic reactions, generally the result of mixing unknown blood types.

Problems with transfusions were not solved until the early twentieth century. In 1900, Viennese pathologist Karl Landsteiner differentiated the four blood types (A, B, AB, and O) based on the presence or absence of certain factors (antigens) on the surface of red blood cells. Dr. Landsteiner developed a method of typing and matching the blood of donors and recipients, for which he was awarded the Nobel Prize. Transfusions of matched blood were performed by sewing the artery of the donor to the vein of the recipient to avoid blood clotting. By World War I, sodium citrate was found to be an effective anticoagulant. That discovery, along with improved refrigeration techniques, gave blood a shelf life for subsequent transfusions.

In 1918, the U.S. Armed Forces endorsed the use of citrated, matched blood as a treatment for hemorrhage and traumatic shock. But problems with mass transportation, storage, and refrigeration made wide-scale transfusions difficult.

The discovery of plasma in the 1930s jump-started the science of transfusions. Plasma is the tea-colored protein liquid of whole blood, separated by centrifuge. It had almost as much therapeutic value as whole blood, but greater versatility. Since plasma did not contain red blood cells, it could be used regardless of blood type. The development of a method to reduce plasma to powdered form, which could be reconstituted with distilled water, revolutionized the transport and storage of blood. Kits containing bottles of plasma and distilled water, along with necessary needles and tubing, were distributed en masse on the battlefields of World War II.

One of the pioneers of plasma development and modern day blood banking was an African American physician, Charles Drew, who established one of the nation's first blood bank programs at New York's Presbyterian Hospital. In 1939, Drew authored "Banked Blood: A Study in Blood Preservation," in which he suggested that plasma could be stored longer than whole blood. The paper became the bible for future blood banks.

War broke out in Europe in 1939. The following year, the Nazis' relentless bombing of London left thousands injured. Blood plasma was in high demand. The head of England's Royal College of Surgeons, a medical school friend of Drew's, requested 5,000 ampules of plasma for Britain. "Blood for Britain" was developed with Drew as its medical director. Operating from New York, he oversaw the first-ever mass mobilization of blood donors, and the first mass production, testing, storage, and shipment of whole blood and plasma. The Transfusion Betterment Association of New York and the American Red Cross assisted with the effort.

By 1941, when the U.S. military was ready to deploy transfusion therapy on the battlefield, it turned to the American Red Cross to provide the massive quantities of blood and plasma required. The Red Cross had had some experience in blood collection. In addition to its role in the Blood for Britain program, a few local chapters had, in the late 1930s, enrolled volunteers willing to donate blood for local hospitals.

The Red Cross complied with the military's request by establishing its first blood collection center in New York City. It hired blood banking expert Dr. Charles Drew as its director. Under Dr. Drew's guidance, the charity recruited donor volunteers, established blood centers, and arranged for the delivery of blood to laboratories for processing into plasma. Red Cross blood centers in large cities were supplemented by bloodmobiles, which cruised suburbs and nearby towns. Each blood center had its monthly quota, based on Army and Navy needs. The blood centers were staffed by a core of professionals, but volunteers were its mainstay.

Eight months into his directorship, Dr. Drew publicly called for an end to the Red Cross policy that segregated the blood of Caucasians and African Americans. The organization was backed by the military and refused to change its mandate. Dr. Drew quit. Red Cross subsequently wrote Charles Drew and the disquieting fact of his race out of its official history for years. His acclaimed Blood for Britain program was termed "not a success" by Red Cross official historian Foster Rhea Dulles.

By 1943, Red Cross's 35 donor centers were logging 76,000 donations a week. In total, 4 million pints of blood would be collected that year. Blood was drawn from donors, sealed in bottles, placed in huge ice coolers, each weighing 400 pounds and storing up to 80 units of blood, and delivered by railroad to the nearest processing center. Special security teams accompanied each shipment to prevent sabotage. At the labs, blood was also spun in large centrifuges to separate plasma, which was further manufactured at the processing center and shipped to military depots and overseas. In California, the Navy set up a supply line for plasma; in less than 48 hours, plasma was traveling from San Francisco through Pearl Harbor or Guam to the battlefront. Plasma was delivered to the frontlines by parachute, landing craft, jeep, and even mules. A *Life* magazine photographer described "combat medics bouncing in jeeps, holding transfusion bottles high as though bearing a torch, shrouded with godlike grace." A Marine correspondent in Iwo Jima cabled home that blood was "the most precious cargo on this island of agony."

The American public responded enthusiastically to those glowing reports from the battlefield. The Red Cross blood donor program fed a vast new industrial machine that produced hundreds of thousands of gallons of plasma, albumin, and pharmaceuticals, which in turn saved thousands of lives. By war's end, Red Cross had provided over thirteen million pints of blood from more than six million volunteer donors.

Civilian demand for blood had meanwhile increased dramatically. Hospitals everywhere were clamoring for blood products. Some formed their own blood banks, others set up organizations to share blood donations. In May 1945, Red Cross national headquarters gave its chapters authority to cooperate with communities to establish blood donor programs.

In 1946, emboldened by the growing demand for blood and conscious of the need to maintain its prominent role in peacetime, the Red Cross unveiled its National Blood Donor Program. Endorsed by the American Medical Association, the American Hospital Association, the U.S. Public Health Service, the Veterans Administration, the Army, and the Navy, the plan called for chapters to initiate Blood Services under the purview of headquarters. Blood would be collected by volunteers and distributed to hospitals or physicians free of charge. Red Cross would recoup only the cost of manufacturing and administering blood products.

A Gallup poll conducted that year found that seventy-three percent of the public favored a national blood program operated by the Red Cross. The *New Republic* hailed National Blood Donor Program as "one of the great humanitarian projects of our time." President Harry S. Truman predicted it would become "the greatest single health activity in history."

The Red Cross plan was not, however, universally embraced. Some county medical societies, local hospitals, and physicians feared competition with hospital blood banks. Others anticipated a Red Cross blood monopoly. In response to these concerns, independent community blood banks and hospital blood banks formed the American Association of Blood Banks (AABB).

The Red Cross National Blood Donor Program was officially launched in 1948. A year later, 28 regional Red Cross blood centers, supported by 500 chapters, supplied blood and plasma to 1,000 hospitals. Local chapters set up collection facilities and recruited donors and volunteers. Headquarters oversaw the collection, processing, and distribution, set policies and standards, and provided funding.

It was not until 1950 and the advent of the Korean War that the Red Cross abandoned its segregation of blood. Blood was in too great a demand for anyone to worry about a donor's race. At that time, the Department of Defense became a partner in the Red Cross blood program and would remain its important supplier and customer. The Red Cross also recognized it could no longer financially sustain its "free blood" service. An expanded cost-recovery system was designed to provide blood to hospitals and other facilities at a fee high enough to cover the cost of processing. The new pricing included a charge for equipment, land, buildings, and working capital.

As its blood program took shape, the Red Cross, led by a group of progressives, adopted a new charter, which was signed into effect by 1947 by President Truman. The old Board of Incorporators and a Central Committee were replaced by a fifty-member Board of Governors, each serving three-year terms. Eight of those members, including the principal officer, or president, were appointed by the President of the United States, who served as honorary Red Cross chair. Membership to the organization was open to all Americans for a fee of one dollar. Special membership categories based on donation amount were abolished.

In 1958, the Red Cross celebrated its seventy-fifth birthday. Roscoe Drummond of the *New York Herald* paid it tribute as "the trustee of the nation's humanity." That year, the Red Cross supplied forty percent of all the blood used in civilian hospitals.

Advancements in technology continued to change the nature of the blood business. Blood could now be separated into red cells, white cells, platelets, and plasma, which in turn could be further broken down into therapeutic components. Red Cross researchers discovered the key to processing fibrinogen, a substance that stopped hemorrhaging. In 1964, the proteins in plasma that helped blood to clot were identified. Red Cross and Hyland Therapeutics Labs, a division of the pharmaceutical firm Baxter Travenol, perfected a method to freeze-dry and bottle a new clotting concentrate called Factor VIII, the protein lacked by hemophiliacs. Thousands afflicted with the disorder became dependent on Factor VIII to control bleeding. The plasma industry's revenues skyrocketed to $1 billion.

The blood and blood products market attracted competitors, but the Red Cross dominated. By the end of the seventies, it was supplying half the nation's blood. The balance of the market was divided between the two nonprofit blood bank groups, the American Association of Blood Banks, which represented about 2,000 hospital and community blood centers, and the Council of Community Blood Centers (CCBC), with 31 regional blood bank members and over 70 independent blood banks. The remainder of the market was supplied by for-profit commercial blood banks, which paid donors twenty-five to fifty dollars per pint.

Rivalry among the blood competitors was often bitter. As the nation's leading charity, whose governing board included Cabinet secretaries and the President of the United States, the Red Cross had a leg up on its nonprofit competitors. Still, the AABB contended that Red Cross was sabotaging its donor recruitment efforts. The AABB's "donor credit" systems which was essential to its community blood drives was a particular target. The AABB gave community blood donors "credits" which could be applied if they or family members required transfusion. In the 1970s the Red Cross denounced the credit system as "profit-making in blood." Meanwhile it, like AABB, charged its hospital clients a processing fee of between $29 and $70 per pint.

Blood shortages and inefficiency in the blood collection and supply system led to further divisiveness. The Red Cross and CCBC established the American Blood Institute to address regional distribution of blood. The American Association of Blood Banks proposed a separate voluntary network of community-based blood banks and transfusion services. The American Blood Resources Association, which represented commercial blood banks and for-profit plasma processing companies, was excluded in the formulation of a national blood program.

Controversy soon erupted over hepatitis, a blood-borne disease that had approached epidemic proportion. By the late 1970s, there was enough hepatitis virus in transfused blood to cause, each year, 30,000 cases of often life-threatening liver disease. Paid donors often were at high risk for transmitting hepatitis. The Red Cross's position was that those paid donors who were frequently drug-users, or habitually diseased, should be eliminated.

In response to the risk of blood-borne hepatitis, the Department of Health, Education and Welfare established, on July 10, 1973, a National Blood Policy. Among its primary goals: making blood accessible to all those in need of transfusion, and maximizing the efficiency and safety of the nation's blood system. Red Cross's strong influence on the resulting policy was apparent. The National Blood Policy called for the adoption of an all-volunteer system for whole blood collection and distribution. Local hospitals were assigned to regional blood collection centers, many of which were operated by the Red Cross. The American Blood Commission, a consortium of the nation's blood banks, was established to implement those objectives. Not surprisingly, the use of paid donor blood dropped sharply. In 1972, paid donors had provided sixteen percent of the nation's blood supply; five years later, the figure was estimated to be between five and ten percent. Officials at the Red Cross thought even that was much too high. "Even if it's only five percent, that's still five hundred thousand bloods," a Red Cross official told the *Washington Post*. "Those five hundred thousand transfusions will cause more hepatitis than the transfusion of five million units of Red Cross volunteer blood."

"Blood collected by commercial blood banks from paid donors is clearly high-risk blood, and we want it labeled," said Dr. Lewellys Barker, blood and blood products director of the Food and Drug Administration (FDA), the agency responsible for regulating the blood industry. By 1978, Dr. Barker would be working for the Red Cross.

Ironically, the Red Cross was also dependent for donations on a population at high risk for hepatitis: sexually active gay men. Homosexual men had participated in studies to develop the hepatitis vaccine; many had stayed on as donors. By the early 1980s, gay and bisexual men would account for about twenty-five percent of the Red Cross donor base.

The Red Cross nonetheless stepped up its lobbying to eliminate paid donor blood from the nation's blood supply. Those efforts were widely perceived as having driven most commercial blood banks out of business and forcing other blood banks to adopt an all-volunteer policy.

By the late 1970s the Red Cross had entered the fast-growing blood products industry, through a lucrative venture with Baxter Travenol Pharmaceutical. The plan was to build a $38 million fractionation plant to manufacture plasma products including albumin and gamma globulin. The Red Cross was already paying commercial labs $9.1 million to produce plasma products, which it sold in 1977 for $29.4 million. With its own processing plant, it intended to double its market share.

That the nonprofit, tax-exempt Red Cross was entering the plasma processing arena using donated blood outraged commercial firms. Should the venture succeed, the Red Cross and Baxter Travenol would control forty-four percent of all plasma collected for fractionation. With sales of $844 million, Baxter Travenol cornered more than twenty-five percent of the plasmapherisis business. Its Fenwal subsidiary dominated ninety percent of the market for blood storage bags, kidney dialysis equipment, and other blood-related supplies.

The nation's independent blood banks accused the blood industry giant of muscling them out of business. Robert Reilly, executive director of the American Blood Resources Association, a trade association representing commercial blood collectors and processors, told *Business Week* in 1978, "We feel the Red Cross is out to eliminate us."

In 1980 the Red Cross entered into an exclusive agreement with Hyland Therapeutics, a division of Baxter Travenol. The new deal would call for a production volume which was four times that of the prior arrangement. By then, Blood Services had become the Red Cross's predominant activity, its biggest revenue generator, earning $244 million, more than half the organization's total revenues. Blood money boosted the Red Cross's overall net worth to nearly half a billion dollars.

Red Cross entered its second century of service with a tribute from President Ronald Reagan. In 1981, Reagan declared March "Red Cross Month," a time "when every citizen is asked to join, serve, and contribute in the same example of the unselfish spirit that characterized the Red Cross since its founding."

CHAPTER FOUR

A BIZARRE ILLNESS

1982

The implication is that the blood was collected from an infected male homosexual.

Dr. Roger Dodd
Assistant Director, Blood Services,
American Red Cross, 1982

On July 9, 1982, Dr. Donald Francis decided that the time had come to make an important phone call. A courageous, impassioned man, he was recognized as someone who functioned well in a crisis—and he had one on his hands: an emerging disease that was probably blood borne.

An epidemiologist, Don Francis tracked epidemics for the Center for Disease Control (the CDC) in Atlanta, Georgia. It was his job to monitor the progress of a disease as it ran its course through a given population. He was also assistant director of the CDC's Division of Viral Diseases. Francis had investigated another blood-borne infection, one that had occurred during the 1970s: hepatitis. A virus that affected the liver, hepatitis had long been a complication faced by patients who had received blood transfusions. A test to detect the presence of hepatitis B surface antigens, which signaled the presence of the disease, had been developed in 1968. Blood collectors routinely used the hepatitis core antibody B test as a screening mechanism. Still, in the mid 1970s, as many as eighteen percent of transfusion recipients were still contracting hepatitis. Subsequently, another infectious culprit was discovered, hepatitis non A–non B.

On this midsummer morning, Francis put a call in to Dr. Roger Dodd, assistant director of Blood Services at the American Red

Cross, and head of its Transmissible Diseases and Immunology Laboratory. Francis and Dodd were both scientists concerned with public health. On that basis, they shared a mutual respect. Francis told Dodd about the imminent publication of the CDC's latest *Morbidity and Mortality Weekly Report (MMWR)*. The lead article of the July 16 issue, Francis said, would be of particular interest to the Red Cross. It concerned what looked like a new illness of potential epidemic proportion, possibly transmitted by blood.

The CDC had recently learned that three hemophiliacs had exhibited a strange syndrome that comprised characteristics of two unusual diseases. One was Kaposi's sarcoma (KS), a skin cancer previously seen only in elderly men of Italian or Jewish descent. KS caused tumors that started on the surface of the skin, then spread to the gastrointestinal and respiratory tracts, resulting in severe internal bleeding. The other an "opportunistic infection" (OI), was *pneumocystis carinii* pneumonia (PCP), an infection of the lungs caused by a single-celled parasite. *Pneumocystis carinii* was generally found only in individuals with impaired immune systems. One of the infected hemophiliacs who had contracted these two illnesses had already died.

The first cases of the disease that would become known as AIDS had been brought to CDC's attention in 1980 by Paul Weizner, head of the Venereal Disease program at the agency. In October of that year, Kaposi's sarcoma had been diagnosed in several young homosexual men in Los Angeles. Thirty-one cases were reported by July 3, 1981 in New York, Los Angeles, and San Francisco. Sensing a unique pathology Weizner alerted his infectious disease colleagues to the possibility of a new disease.

Paralleling these developments in immune disorders was an increase in requests made to CDC for pentamidine, a prescription drug used to treat PCP. The drug was manufactured by a British company; it was not licensed for sale in the United States. CDC had the authority to dispense pentamidine, but only if all other treatments had failed. The sudden demand had caught the eye of Dr. Bruce Evatt, CDC's director of the Division of Host Factors and head of the agency's hematology department. Evatt had received a call from a physician in Florida whose hemophilia patient had died of PCP. The doctor speculated that the PCP had been transmitted through the Factor VIII clotting concentrate his patient had been prescribed. Evatt told him that was impossible. He had never seen PCP in a hemophiliac. Nonetheless, Evatt began to look for other cases.

He would later describe the pentamidine files as a "godsend."

While Evatt began a watch on CDC's pentamidine files, his colleague Dr. James Curran was tracking the disease among homosexual men, Haitians, and IV drug users. Francis received his first call about KS/OI from Curran. The two men had worked together years earlier developing the hepatitis B vaccine. They had conducted studies in gay men in Los Angeles and were familiar with infectious disease paradigms and risks associated with sexual behavior common in the gay community. Curran's description of KS/OI intrigued Francis. When he began investigating the disorder, Francis immediately observed striking similarities to hepatitis, which was profoundly troublesome. If this disease were blood borne, its containment could be problematic.

Francis had earned his post-doctorate in virology and infectious disease at Harvard. He was also an expert in feline leukemia, an immnosuppressive disease in cats. On a hunch, he pulled out his cat studies. Combine feline leukemia and hepatitis, Francis told Curran, and you've got KS/OI.

In July 1981, CDC established its KS Task Force, headed by Curran, to monitor and investigate cases of opportunistic infections. CDC had also begun designing a case/control study to examine the epidemiology of what was then referred to as Gay Related Immunodeficiency (GRID), because of its prevalence in the homosexual community. Antibodies in sperm and a sexual enhancement drug known as "poppers" (amyl nitrate) were initially suspected as the causal agents.

By June, 1982, the disease had claimed 355 victims, including heterosexuals. In July, CDC learned that three hemophiliacs exhibited the immune disorder. All were white, heterosexual men with no history of IV drug use. All had used Factor VIII during the prior five years.

Hemophilia is a rare inherited disorder that affects only males. It is caused by a genetic deficiency of a particular blood protein that aids clotting. About sixty percent of hemophiliacs suffer the most extreme form of the disease: spontaneous bleeding into multiple joints and muscles. It can be fatal. To remedy this lack of blood-clotting protein, hemophiliacs rely on either a product derived from fresh frozen plasma (cryoprecipitate) or, more commonly, a protein concentrate prepared from these precipitates called antihemophiliac factor, (AHF) or Factor VIII. Factor VIII was developed in 1968 by researchers at the Red Cross and Hyland Therapeutics. It was mass produced by pooling plasma from about 20,000 donors, then drawing off the proteins that caused blood to clot. The average paid donor gave about 40 to 60 times a year. Thus a significant number of plasma pools could be contaminated by a few diseased donors. Since the average hemophiliac used between 50,000 and 100,000 units of Factor VIII each year, he was particularly vulnerable to any pathogen in the blood supply.

The dispersion of the opportunistic infection among hemophiliacs clinched it for Francis. His suspicions about blood were underscored by CDC's official report later that month: "The clinical and immunologic features these three patients share are strikingly similar to those recently observed among certain individuals from the following groups: homosexual males, heterosexual IV drug users and Haitians. Although the cause of the severe immune dysfunction is unknown, the occurrence of three cases among hemophiliacs suggests the possible transmission of an agent through blood products."

The mortality rate for KS/OI was then 67 percent. If the disease were blood borne, not only hemophiliacs but as many as four to six million people who, for various medical reasons, needed some form of blood product every year were in mortal danger.

The small number of cases were, Francis believed, a mere intimation of what was to come, the proverbial "tip of the epidemiological iceberg." But it was going to be difficult to convince the public they were in the middle of an epidemic if they could not see its manifestations. KS/OI was not going to be like smallpox, which Francis had tracked and helped eradicate in the early 1970s in Yugoslavia, India, and Bangladesh. KS/OI was not like the exotic Ebola virus, either. He had seen Ebola close up in the Sudan in 1976, as a member of a World Health Organization team investigating the first outbreak of African hemorrhagic fever. Ebola broke fast and ugly, killing several hundred people in one fell swoop. Then it disappeared. KS/OI, with its suspected long incubation period, was a slow burner. Dramatic symptoms might not appear in the general population for years. Meanwhile, asymptomatic carriers were having sex, giving blood, and living their lives.

KS/OI's epidemiological similarity to hepatitis was so striking that before calling Dodd, Francis sent a memo to Jim Curran urging him to "rapidly investigate" KS/OI's potential transmission by blood or blood products. He recommended a four-point strategy that included surveillance of hemophiliacs and transfusion-associated cases. This would involve determining which gay men frequented high-risk bath houses and had donated blood. Recipients of this blood would then be traced. Francis also proposed a survey of large numbers of blood donors to determine their sexual preference, followed by a traceback of recipients of blood donated by male homosexuals.

"In the absence of solid recommendations," Don Francis warned, "lives could be lost."

Bruce Evatt had also sent a similar alert to Mount Sinai Medical Center's Dr. Louis Aledort, chairman of the National Hemophilia Foundation. "We have been suspicious," Evatt wrote, "that [KS/OI] may be transmitted in a manner similar to hepatitis, and thus creates a problem for users of blood products."

CDC's capability to deal with the enormity of a blood-borne epidemic was limited. Its federal budget had been slashed fifteen percent, in part due to the Reagan administration's official position that all infectious diseases in the U.S. had been eradicated, or at least were under control. CDC had recently been granted only $400,000 to investigate KS/OI.

Don Francis thought it reasonable to ask Dodd for the Red Cross's help in designing and implementing KS studies. The Red Cross would have a distinct interest, Francis thought, in blood safety. At that point, the American Red Cross was collecting half the blood in the United States, approximately six million units of whole blood from about four million voluntary donors. That amounted to about twenty thousand blood collections every working day of the year.

Francis's prior experiences with the Red Cross had been relatively straightforward. He figured he would "give them the grain and the oats and they'd go galloping."

So on the morning of July 9, Francis called his former research colleague and told him about the potentially lethal dangers to the blood supply from this new immunodeficiency syndrome. Francis explained that KS/OI appeared to share at least one of the routes of transmission of hepatitis and that the three hemophiliac cases most likely indicated a blood-borne agent. The donor, Francis told Dodd, had been an infected male homosexual.

Francis said he was concerned about the Red Cross's policy of accepting active male homosexuals.

The news that blood might transmit a fatal disease associated with the gay lifestyle boded ill for the Red Cross. The blood banker relied on gay men for about fifteen percent of its donations. By 1982, blood had become the Red Cross's leading revenue generator. Blood services would, by year end, earn about $371 million, up $70 million from 1981. After expenses, the profit margin on blood enabled the organization to boost its 1982 earnings nearly $44 million above the prior year.

After speaking with Francis, Roger Dodd sent a confidential memo to Dr. Alfred Katz. As executive director of the Red Cross's Blood Services, Fred Katz was responsible for the administration and management of Blood Services and blood collection at its then fifty-seven blood centers. Dodd conveyed to Katz the content of his conversation with Don Francis. "The major causes for alarm," Dodd wrote, "are the mortality of the disease complex and its apparent infectious nature. Because of the unusual rarity of this disease and because it does appear to share at least one of the routes of transmission of hepatitis B, a number of epidemiologists have suggested that the three cases discussed, represent blood-borne transmission of the agent(s) involved. The implication is that the blood was collected from an infected male homosexual."

Dodd indicated that this connection was "clearly speculative" but that it had "led to specific concerns about accepting active male homosexuals as blood donors," a group that was at higher risk for hepatitis B infection. As a result of these concerns, the National Center for Drugs and Biologics planned to convene an expert panel to address this issue. Dodd suggested that the Red Cross establish a working group to develop policy relating to blood donations from active male homosexuals.

On July 6, Dr. William Foege, CDC director and Assistant Surgeon General at the Department of Health and Human Services, sent a memo to Hemophilia Treatment Centers and state and territorial epidemiologists alerting them to the three hemophilia cases. Foege pointed out that the cause of the immune dysfunction was unknown. However, he noted, "the possibility of a transmissible agent has been suggested and concern about possible transmission through blood products has been raised." Ten days later, a Public Health Service meeting was held to discuss the risks to the blood supply. The mode of transmission was becoming apparent; that is, blood seemed to be a vehicle. At the meeting, Under Secretary for Health Dr. Edward Brandt formed a PHS task force of scientists from FDA, CDC and NIH. They would review critical information concerning the hemophilia cases and make recommendations. The task force's first meeting was scheduled for July 27.

Nonetheless, on July 21, the American Red Cross, which would send delegates to that PHS meeting, issued the following statement to its blood regions: "There is no data available to us to suggest that the underlying disease or associated conditions are transmitted by blood." Ominously, the statement continued, "No change is indicated at this time in current practices regarding donor recruitment or screening."

At the July 27 PHS meeting of the Committee on Opportunistic Infection in Hemophiliacs, Dr. Gerald Sandler, associate director of medical and laboratory services, represented the Red Cross. Sandler's primary responsibility was to provide medical opinion on Blood Services policies to Red Cross management. He also supervised its testing laboratories in Bethesda and Rockville, Maryland. The Red Cross had been asked to attend the PHS meeting, since, apart from blood collection, it also provided plasma for the manufacture of hemophilia clotting factor.

The appearance of PCP in the three hemophiliacs was particularly worrisome. As the meeting's minutes reflected, "If the PCP observed in three patients with hemophilia represents the same process as seen in other groups with AIDS, then a possible mode of transmission is via blood products."

The meeting was Sandler's first introduction to the disease that would, that day, be named Acquired Immune Deficiency Syndrome (AIDS). He recalled that participants acknowledged that AIDS displayed characteristics suggesting an infectious agent, most likely a virus. The participants also concurred that the risks of certain blood products, particularly Factor VIII, should be examined.

Sandler left that meeting thinking that AIDS might be blood borne. He was not convinced, however, that gay men should refrain from donating blood.

That day, the PHS made several suggestions to blood collectors. These included establishing an active surveillance system to determine whether other suspicious cases of AIDS were occurring in hemophiliac patients; detailed lab studies; and devising practical ways to decrease or eliminate the infectious risks from Factor VIII.

However, no mandate or order compelling blood bankers to act upon these suggestions was issued by the PHS or the FDA.

Shortly after that meeting, Dr. Dennis Donohue, director of the Division of Blood and Blood Products at FDA, asked Cutter Laboratories, a leading manufacturer of Factor VIII, to *voluntarily* exclude plasma collected from known homosexuals. An internal Cutter

memo indicated that Donohue was "not basing this request on scientific concerns that such plasma transmits AIDS, but because it was
believed that the action was a political necessity to prevent national
adverse publicity and undue concerns in the hemophiliac population."

Dennis Donohue was a former blood banker. In the 1960s he had
been director of the King County Central Blood Bank in Washington State, then went on to become executive director of the Puget
Sound Blood Center. Prior to joining FDA's Division of Blood and
Blood Products, Donohue had served as chairman of the Red Cross
Medical Advisory Committee. He was now responsible for all scientific, regulatory activities relating to blood and blood products, including licensing of blood establishments, and approval of
procedures, inspections and tests used in blood product processing,
such as hepatitis B core antibody.

FDA's blood chief worked closely with the Blood Products Advisory Council. BPAC was established in 1980 to make recommendations to FDA concerning blood safety. It was comprised largely of
blood industry representatives who suggested to FDA how it should
run the blood business—which standards to require, what regulations to mandate and enforce. This self-monitoring reflected FDA's
view that blood bankers were benign stewards of the public health
who had no interest, financial or otherwise, to do the public wrong.

In August, 1982—one month after the PHS meeting—the ever-
vigilant CDC learned of a curious case of an elderly Connecticut
woman who had recently died of immune suppression. The case
caught the attention of Dr. Dale Lawrence, a CDC medical officer
in Atlanta. Lawrence had been tracking incidences of immune suppression disease among recipients of blood. In all cases to date, at
least one high-risk donor had been implicated. Suspecting a transfusion-AIDS case, Lawrence contacted the hospital that had reported
her death. The attending physician informed him that the woman
had undergone successful breast surgery. To the best of his knowledge, she had not received blood transfusions.

Lawrence left his mind open to other possibilities. Perhaps the patient had had a secret life; perhaps her ex-husband had. But
Lawrence turned up nothing to contradict the profile of a staid, conservative matron. He persevered and gained access to the surgery
records. Buried within reams of charts was what he was looking for:
two slips of paper indicating that the woman had received several
units of blood.

The blood had come from a Red Cross center in Connecticut.

The Red Cross was willing to provide Lawrence with the names of the two blood donors involved—names only; no phone numbers, no addresses. The blood banker expressed concern about donor confidentiality, and Lawrence knew he was up against the classic "catch-22." The blood banks wanted proof from CDC that AIDS was blood borne, yet they would offer limited assistance in tracing infected donors.

Lawrence had a hunch about one of the donors. It took some riffling through phone books and dozens of calls, but he managed to locate the donor's mother. She told him that her son had some emotional problems associated with his lifestyle; she did not or could not elaborate. He had, she said, moved to Columbus, Ohio.

Lawrence rallied his state health agency contacts and the donor was found. He appeared very agitated but agreed to be interviewed. In that session, Dale Lawrence learned what the Red Cross blood intake staff had not. Prior to giving blood in Connecticut, the young man had had unprotected sex with two high-risk women: one injected drugs, the other was a Haitian. The donor agreed to a blood test. A T-cell test assessed his immune system response as indicative of a pattern associated with AIDS.

Years later Lawrence would recall his frustration in dealing with the Red Cross: "We felt extremely thwarted doing our job to protect public health, which was to search far back up the trail to ascertain donor risks. We didn't like skulking around, but the Red Cross was more concerned about the civil rights of donors than the larger public health imperative." Lawrence had begun to wonder whether "vested interests" on the part of blood bankers had superseded the public's welfare, but he was particularly disillusioned with the Red Cross. "People tend to look at that organization as standing for the epitome of care and responsibility, to be the leader that could have taken a leadership role—but they didn't."

The Connecticut transfusion AIDS case was cited months later in a memo which Red Cross blood director Fred Katz sent to four colleagues: vice president Lewellys Barker; Joseph O'Malley, Gerald Sandler; and Roger Dodd. Katz told them that Connecticut Red Cross had given the names of two donors to CDC. "I'm not sure how follow-up took place," Katz wrote. "Dr. Currin [sic] said that one donor is in Connecticut and is healthy, the other moved to Ohio. At the time of donation he was healthy, but [was since] hospitalized with a 'bizarre illness'."

In that same correspondence, Katz reported that CDC had identified 636 cases of AIDS. About 20 to 25 were not members of risk groups; for 3 of these people, their only risk factor had been a blood transfusion. Katz told Barker, O'Malley, Sandler and Dodd, that James Curran was convinced "that AIDS is a result of a transmissible agent, that it is transmissible by blood, that gay individuals should be excluded from blood donation, and that the impact on the blood supply should be studied now by organizations like ours."

Subsequently, Roger Dodd wrote to a colleague, "We have indeed become very interested, although not functionally active, in the whole issue of AIDS." The epidemiological pattern of the syndrome did suggest "some sort of blood-borne etiologic agent."

On November 2, Barker received an urgent letter from Louis Aledort of the National Hemophilia Foundation. Five cases of AIDS among hemophiliacs had been "confirmed," he wrote. Other cases were under review by CDC. Aledort expressed concern that AIDS "may be an infectious agent transmitted by high-risk population groups to hemophiliacs through blood products." The NHF had passed a resolution "in view of the potential risk of transmission [of AIDS] by transfusion of blood products . . . to urge all sources of Factor VIII products to exclude from plasma donations all individuals" who belong to high-risk groups: homosexuals, IV drug users, and those who recently resided in Haiti. Aledort wanted Barker's comments and suggestions concerning "the feasability of expanding donor restrictions."

In early December 1982, a meeting of the FDA's Blood Products Advisory Committee was hastily convened at the National Library of Medicine in Bethesda, Maryland. At the time, BPAC's acting chairman was Dr. William V. Miller, then director of the American Red Cross's Blood Services for the Missouri-Illinois region. Over sandwiches, Miller listened to a presentation given by CDC's Dr. Bruce Evatt. Evatt told his audience that the epidemic was rising at an almost exponential pace. There were 788 domestic cases and about 50 foreign which had been reported since mid-1979; Evatt told attendees that the epidemiologic pattern of AIDS seems to be similar to that of hepatitis. "Cases are now appearing among contacts of persons in the high risk groups." Eight hemophiliacs who had received clotting factor had contracted AIDS. About five cases of AIDS had been reported to CDC in the prior eighteen months in patients who had had blood transfusions. Evatt told his audience that one donor was later diagnosed with AIDS.

Transfusion-AIDS could follow the same increasing pattern seen with hemophiliac patients, he said.

It was highly probable, Evatt stated, that AIDS had already made inroads into the nation's blood supply. As the CDC official would later testify in a lawsuit brought by HIV infected hemophiliacs, "You didn't have to be a rocket scientist in mid-1982 to strongly suspect AIDS was blood borne."

What Evatt said at the BPAC meeting impressed Miller. "It seemed," Miller would later recall, "we had the makings of a new disease that was probably transmissible, whether by blood or not. What we did have was a terrible disease which looked as though it was going to take a very heavy toll on the American people."

Miller also recognized the makings of a political bombshell.

Despite the vulnerability of the nation's blood supply, BPAC did not suggest to the blood industry that it defer high-risk donors. The subject was barely mentioned by the advisory board to the FDA, although the meeting records indicate "a sense of urgency because of the continuing spread of AIDS and because of its long incubation period." The FDA's Dennis Donohue stated at the meeting that high-risk donor exclusion "is not subject to responsible regulatory action. I think that the voluntary blood banking organizations must look at the question, remembering their responsibility for the blood supply and their basic social responsibility."

Shortly after the BPAC meeting, Red Cross's Fred Katz received drafts from Jim Curran and Bruce Evatt of two articles scheduled for the December 10 issue of CDC's *Morbidity and Mortality Weekly Report.* The first article reviewed the cases of four hemophiliacs diagnosed with AIDS-related opportunistic infections. Another suspected AIDS case, a seven-year-old hemophiliac in Los Angeles, was under investigation.

The second article described an unexplained immunodeficiency in a twenty-month-old baby born prematurely in San Francisco in March 1981. During his one-month hospital stay, he had received nineteen blood transfusions, including whole blood, packed red blood cells, and platelets. When discharged, the child appeared to be healthy. Six months later, he began showing signs of an immune disfunction.

An investigation into the source of the child's transfusion indicated that one of the donors had subsequently been diagnosed with AIDS. The forty-six-year-old homosexual donor had been asymptomatic in March 1981, when he donated blood. A year later he was dead.

CDC reported: "If platelet transfusion contained an etiologic [causative] agent for AIDS, one must assume that the agent can be present in the blood of a donor before onset of symptomatic illness and that the incubation period for such illness can be relatively long. This model for AIDS transmission is consistent with findings described in an investigation of a cluster of sexually related AIDS cases among homosexual men in southern California."

For Red Cross officials Gerald Sandler and general counsel Karen Shoos Lipton, the infant's case was a turning point, the first documentation they had seen of what was now termed transfusion AIDS. Lipton would later tell government investigators, "The light gradually dawned."

In a December 7, 1982, memo sent to Arnie deBeaufort, head of a newly formed Red Cross AIDS working group, Sandler wrote: "The evidence that acquired immunodeficiency syndrome (AIDS) is caused by a transmissible agent is increasing, but the data is still not sufficiently conclusive to actually initiate donor deferral practices at this time. On the other hand, it may be prudent, necessary, to do so at some future time, potentially as early as six–eight weeks from now. Surely Blood Services should discourage all regional Blood Services from specifically recruiting gay donors."

The inevitability of eliminating as many as 15 percent of the Red Cross's repeat donors, without publicly acknowledging the dangers to the blood supply, would require delicate maneuvering. It was, as Dr. William Miller of the Red Cross had earlier pointed out to his BPAC colleagues, "like dancing on the head of a pin."

There were two possible options for culling out these gay donors without implicating their sexual orientation or the safety of Red Cross blood. Sandler suggested that blood intake nurses could assess the donor's confidential history to determine his suitability. Another option was providing gay donors with sufficient information on AIDS which should allow them to exclude themselves, i.e. "self deferral."

Like many of Sandler's colleagues, Dr. Peter Page, chief medical director of the Red Cross's Northeast Region, supported self deferral. Page also had recently learned of an impending CDC meeting during which blood was going to be formally, and publicly, implicated. He decided to contact Fred Katz with a donor screening proposal which would show that the Red Cross was acting in good faith. In a December 16 confidential memo to Katz, Page suggested subtle changes in the Red Cross donor deferral system. The focus should be "donors likely to be at significant risk without singling out only the gay male population. Accordingly we would not then need to change our criteria as the epidemic spreads to transfusion recipients, health care providers, female sex partners of intravenous drug abusers, household contacts of AIDS carriers, etc."

The following day Fred Katz received yet another missive urging the Red Cross take action. Dr. Joseph Bove, chairman of the American Association of Blood Banks' Committee on Transfusion Transmitted Diseases, informed Katz that he was compelled to call an urgent meeting. The time had come for the industry to create a uniform policy for dealing with transfusion AIDS. The Red Cross, the American Association of Blood Banks and the Council of Community Blood Centers needed to present a "relatively uniform posture." United, they must develop a common standard for industry practices during this crisis.

"I think it is fair to say," Bove wrote, "that the more one learns about AIDS, the more concerned one becomes about the potential for major problems in the blood collecting sector . . . My current best guess is that we are dealing with an infectious agent able to be spread by blood and blood products and that individuals who receive large quantities of Factor concentrate are at an increased risk. I think we are under great pressure to do 'anything and everything' to curtail the spread of AIDS."

Bove told Katz that he would draft a basic policy statement which the Red Cross could then develop. "We can, with any luck, have something fairly well settled before the end of our meeting . . . so that those of you with early flights can get out of Washington in good time."

CHAPTER FIVE

THRESHOLD OF DEATH

1983

AIDS is transmissible by blood.

Dr. Joseph O'Malley
Office of Product Development and Clinical Evaluation
The American Red Cross

CDC had decided to call a meeting at the beginning of 1983 to discuss new developments concerning AIDS and gain a better understanding of the disease. The evidence was mounting that transmission occurred through person-to-person contact and blood products. Recent PHS studies had shown T-cell ratio abnormalities, an indication of immunosuppression, among many hemophiliacs who had received clotting factor. By the first of the year, 30 to 50 percent of all hemophiliacs in the U.S. were displaying immune system problems. More than 700 cases of AIDS had been reported to CDC since 1982; about 70 percent were homosexual males. In hemophiliacs, five cases of AIDS had been confirmed and three more were highly suspect.

AIDS appeared to have at least a one-year incubation period, which would account for the low numbers of reported cases.

For many recipients of blood products, Don Francis realized, it was already too late. Nonetheless he looked forward to the CDC meeting. The agency could assist the blood bankers in formulating an action plan that could stem the transmission of AIDS through the blood supply.

For one, blood bankers must begin asking male donors about their sexual lifestyle. Specifically, if they had ever had sex with a man.

CDC officials were more concerned about the blood bankers' response to a preventive measure that could cost them money. Namely, the use of a surrogate test to screen out high-risk candidates for AIDS. There was no specific blood test for AIDS, but the hepatitis B core antibody test (anti HBc) showed a significant degree of accuracy in identifying donors who were at high risk for AIDS. CDC's top virologist, Thomas Spira, found that 90 percent of patients with AIDS were positive for hepatitis core antibodies. Spira had determined that 88 percent of known cases of AIDS among homosexual men showed the presence of the antibodies.

In the absence of an AIDS-specific serologic marker, the hepatitis core antibody was, CDC determined, the best interim measure.

Anticipating blood bankers' concerns about cost, CDC had done some price checking. The test would price out at two to five dollars per unit of donated blood, an amount that could easily be deflected onto hospital clients.

Still, Don Francis and Bruce Evatt expected resistance. The industry had historically dragged its heels in accepting and implementing new procedures, whether that meant additional blood tests or minor changes in how they did their paperwork. Such resistance to change seemed, to Francis, to be characteristic of the kind of individual who went into blood banking. These were not epidemic busters. In his experience, blood bankers were orderly traditionalists who were comfortable with the status quo. In Bruce Evatt's opinion, blood bankers were simply business people concerned with issues of supply and demand.

However, AIDS had precipitated a crisis situation. Blood bankers would have to adopt an uncharacteristic persona: they would have to become agents of change.

Evatt and Francis expected some resistance. They did not expect war.

Nearly 200 people attended the January 4, 1983 "Workshop to Identify Opportunities for Prevention of Acquired Immune Deficiency Syndrome" in Atlanta. Many, like Gerald Sandler and Paul Cumming of the Red Cross, had participated in the July 27 session held by the PHS, as had hemophilia experts, the American Association of Blood Banks, and the Council of Community Blood Banks. Also present at the January meeting were representatives from the American Blood Commission, the Irwin Memorial Blood Center in San Francisco, the National Gay Task Force, the Pharmaceutical Manufacturers Association, and the New York City

Health Department, as well as officials from the FDA, the CDC, and the NIH.

Dr. Joseph Bove, chairman of the industry's Committee on Transfusion Transmitted Disease and chair of the BPAC, would later characterize the meeting as a "Roman circus."

The tension was palpable among the various factions. CDC and FDA were not on the best of terms. Mistrust and rivalry had festered between the two agencies for years. Friction was stoked in the mid-1970s, when CDC had recommended a massive immunization program to combat the swine flu epidemic. Millions had been innoculated, but adverse reaction to the vaccine had caused some deaths. This episode would diminish FDA confidence in CDC's warnings about yet another epidemic. Many at FDA believed that CDC was meddling in issues that only the regulatory agency should address.

Evatt opened the meeting by reviewing recent CDC data concerning risks groups, and blood and plasma donation. He told attendees the death of the twenty-month-old infant in San Francisco was unequivocally a result of blood donated by a gay man infected with AIDS. In the other cases, gay donors had also been implicated.

Tom Spira proceeded with the epidemiological evidence that surrogate tests showed a high correlation between hepatitis B and AIDS. Using such a test, potentially high-risk donors could be efficiently and objectively eliminated from the donor pool. The tests were, Spira said, "highly sensitive and highly specific."

Tom Drees, owner of Alpha Pharmaceutical, a manufacturer of clotting factor, was stunned at what he heard. "I was," he later told *Frontline*, "literally knocked off my chair. [They said,] "Here's this new disease. It's blood borne. It's a retrovirus, we think. It's doubling every six months, and it's a hundred percent fatal." As far as he was concerned, you didn't have to be an epidemiologist to know you had to do something fast. When Drees told his colleagues he was going to initiate stringent screening procedures, they said he was crazy. "I had one group say to me, 'You're going to turn a donor down, he's going to walk out the door, down the street, come into my place, and we'll take him all day long. You're a sucker. You're a jerk for doing this.' Well, sorry. That's the way we see it."

The subsequent discussion among blood bankers quickly degenerated into arguments about whether transfusion AIDS existed at all. The National Hemophilia Foundation suggested that AIDS in hemophiliacs was simply the result of a "lifetime exposure to immune complexes"; it had nothing to do with allegedly HIV-infected blood. Hyland Labs, which was under contractual agreement to distribute Red Cross plasma, objected to surrogate testing as too exclusionary and costly.

Bruce Voeller, executive director of the National Gay Task Force, saw the issue as one of cost. Voeller would tell *Frontline*, "The volunteer industry was particularly strongly and adamantly opposed to using the hepatitis B core antibody test as surrogate test for screening out infected blood because of the cost. It was as simple as that. It was, from their point of view, going to add a great deal to their costs and loss of their profits."

It was the Red Cross's position that direct questioning of gay males was an unacceptable infringement of privacy and civil rights. As Sandler would later testify in Roland Ray's transfusion-AIDS lawsuit, "Direct or indirect questions about a person's sexual preference are inappropriate. Such an invasion of privacy can be justified only if it demonstrates clear-cut benefit." No such benefit was apparent to the Red Cross in 1983. "We had a system that was working, 40,000 units of blood a day were being collected, and they were just about barely meeting the needs of people who were bleeding and needed blood for transfusion." As to whether the Red Cross should have restricted donations from gay men, or asked directly about high-risk sexual behavior, Sandler explained, "Those questions, no matter how well intentioned, were ineffective in eliminating those donors who might carry AIDS."

As Don Francis listened to blood bankers alternately debate civil rights, cost, and whether AIDS even existed, he was dumbstruck. He later recalled, "The blood industry did not want to put health in front of trouble. But this was more than blindsightedness. This was reckless endangerment."

Francis could no longer restrain himself. He stood up and slammed his fist against the conference table. "How many people have to die?" he shouted. "Just tell us how many people have to die. Ten, twenty, forty? Let's stop the meeting right now, and you give us the threshold of death you need before you believe this is really happening. We'll meet at that time so we can start talking about doing something."

By the end of the day the blood bankers had reached a consensus. They agreed it was desirable to exclude high-risk donors to reduce the transmission of AIDS by blood. But no one could agree on just how that would be accomplished.

Francis expressed his anger and frustration to Dr. Jeff Koplan, assistant director at CDC, days after the meeting. "I feel there is a strong possibility that some post-transfusion AIDS and much post–Factor VIII receipt of AIDS will occur in this country in the coming two years," Francis wrote. "For hemophiliacs, I fear it might be too late." He urged Koplan to issue strong recommendations, which would undoubtedly be "controversial" to blood bankers. "But to wait for the blood bankers to approve our recommendations will only endanger the public's health."

William Foege was also convinced that the immunosuppression underlying AIDS was caused by an agent that could be transmitted through intimate person-to-person contact as well as by blood and blood products. In a letter to CDC officials after the meeting, Foege wrote, "The possibility of acquiring AIDS through transfusion of blood from an AIDS donor is suggested by several cases." He advised that donor screening, including lab tests, "should be evaluated for their effectiveness in identifying and excluding blood of high-risk donors."

On January 6, as Francis bemoaned the industry's inertia and Foege acknowledged the dangers to blood recipients, the Red Cross participated in the first meeting of the American Association of Blood Banks Committee on Transfusion Transmitted Diseases. The outcome of that gathering was a policy statement, which would be released on January 13. That statement established, literally overnight, the industry's "standard of care." If the blood bankers were to follow the statement guidelines, they could not, they theorized, be held liable should their analysis of the AIDS situation later prove incorrect. Gerald Sandler described the process by which the "Joint Statement on Acquired Immune Deficiency Syndrome Related to Transfusions" was created as a way the three blood organizations had "of trying to put our heads together, come up with what we thought was the best scientific evidence, put it in writing, disseminate it, and let everyone out there see what we were thinking."

In one unified voice, the Red Cross and its peers decided, "The predominant mode of transmission seems to be from person to person, probably involving intimate contact. The possibility of blood-borne spread, still unproven, has been raised, an impression reinforced by eight confirmed cases in hemophiliacs treated with AHF concentrate and by a case in a newborn infant who received nineteen units of blood components, one of which was from a donor who later died of AIDS." Still, "No agent has been isolated and there is no test for the disease or for potential carriers. Evidence for transmission by blood transfusion is inconclusive at this time."

The blood bankers decided their major effort should revolve around two areas: "1. additional caution in the use of blood and blood products; and 2. reasonable attempts to limit blood donations from individuals or groups that may have an unacceptably high risk of AIDS." To that end, they were going to undertake educational campaigns, encourage autologous (self-donated) donations; prepare to deal with requests for Factor VIII alternatives; and make changes in donor screening. This new screening approach would involve asking donors questions "to detect possible AIDS or exposure to patients with AIDS." Those questions focused on symptoms, not lifestyle.

The statement continued, "The presently available medical and scientific evidence that AIDS can be spread by blood components remains incomplete. Should evidence of a clearly implicated donor population become apparent, specific recommendations . . . will be made promptly. [Despite] considerable pressure on the blood banking community to restrict blood donations by gay males, direct or indirect questions about a donor's sexual preference are inappropriate. There is reason to believe that such questions, no matter how well intentioned, are ineffective in eliminating those donors who many carry AIDS."

As for surrogate testing: "We do not advise routine implementation of any laboratory screening program for AIDS at this time."

Dr. Joseph Bove, of the Committee on Transfusion Transmitted Diseases reported on January 21, 1983, to his Committee members, including the Red Cross, that an additional child with AIDS has been admitted to a Texas hospital. The child had, at birth, received seven blood transfusions, one of which came from an AIDS-infected donor. "This case increases the probability that AIDS may be spread by blood. Furthermore, the CDC continues to investigate the current cases aggressively and may even have a few more. While I believe our report reacts appropriately to the data at hand, I also believe that the most we can do in this situation is buy time. There is little doubt in my mind that additional transfusion-related cases and additional cases in patients with hemophilia will surface.

"We will be obliged to review our current stance and probably to move in the same direction as the commercial fractionators. By that

I mean, it will be essential for us to take some active steps to screen out donor populations who are at high risk of AIDS. For practical purposes, this means gay males. . . .

"We are reluctant to do this since we do not want anything that we do now to be interpreted by social (or by legal) authorities as agreeing with the concept—as yet unproven—that AIDS can be spread by blood."

Despite the implacable official stance the Red Cross showed the public, AIDS and its threat to the blood supply profoundly disturbed the blood banker. To concede that blood was in danger, let alone by a disease affecting gay men, would deal a severe blow to its pristine image of capable stewardship. To abstain from action might precipitate an epidemic. Fred Katz decided to survey his key staffers for their opinion about what should be done. On January 26, Red Cross Blood Services director sent a confidential memo to sixteen Blood Services officers. In it he posed several questions: Is AIDS transmissible by blood? Will elimination of donor groups at risk decrease incidence? Should we eliminate those groups? If so, how?

Within a period of several days, Katz received replies via Arnie de-Beaufort of the Red Cross AIDS Task Force. In memos dated February 1, 1983, Drs. Joseph O'Malley and Gerald Sandler expressed concern about blood-borne AIDS. Sandler wrote that AIDS was "possibly" transmitted by blood, but that "scientific evidence is not conclusive." Eliminating high-risk donors would "not necessarily" reduce AIDS in the blood supply. O'Malley believed that "AIDS is transmissible by blood."

Victor Schmitt, associate director of Plasma Products Management, answered that "it would appear likely" that AIDS is transmissible by blood and that eliminating high-risk donors would probably decrease incidence of AIDS in the blood.

His colleague Dr. J. B. Schorr responded that "AIDS very probably is a transmissible disorder. In the cases of a parent-child transfusion or transmission among IV drug users, blood seems likely to be the vehicle." Was it "at all likely" that AIDS could be blood-transmitted? "The answer to this question is certainly 'Yes,' and much of what I believe Red Cross Blood Services ought to do is based on that possibility. The approach which says 'we will do nothing until it is positively proved that blood is a vehicle for transmission of AIDS' could do considerable harm to a few blood recipients, and to the Red Cross image."

Schorr's advice was clear: "We should strive to eliminate, to the extent possible, high-risk donors, and we should do it now. The major justification is that their blood may be infectious. AIDS is a letal disease, and it is incumbent upon blood suppliers to minimize the risk of its transmission, even at the expense of embarrassing a portion of the donor population. . . . if it turns out to be a viral disease transmissible by blood and we have held back, it will not soon be forgotten."

But even Schorr demurred from advocating direct questioning. "Direct questioning of all male donors in all parts of the USA seems," he posited, "overly enthusiastic."

Schorr's optimistic forbearance was based on a perception that permeated the upper echelons of the Red Cross: that there were "fast-lane" gays and then there were those who were benignly "in the closet." This philosophy was also articulated by statistician Paul Cumming. In addressing Katz's question, "Is AIDS transmissible by blood?" Cumming wrote, "The available evidence strongly suggests that "AIDS is transmissible;" [it is] "transmissible via AHF concentrate to hemophiliacs;" but, he added, there was "not enough evidence to draw any other scientific conclusion" [emphasis in original].

"Scientifically," Cumming observed, "we don't know, since the transmission mechanism is unknown at present. In the future, however, it is likely to be shown that such will be the case." In the meantime the issue was "ethical/political/marketing/legal."

From the marketing standpoint, Cumming noted that "we will be better off making direct and visible attempt at elimination of such groups. Ethically I don't think sexual preference is the proper business of anyone (or any institution) other than the individuals involved in the sexual act."

Cumming explained that while homosexuals and bisexuals constituted up to 25 percent of the Red Cross's donor population, with male homosexuals equaling "15 percent or less" of those donors, only a "small subset of gays are those associated with AIDS, the so-called 'fast-lane' or 'bath house' gays. Eliminating those gays probably would not be noticeable."

As far as he could determine, the Red Cross was facing a "lose-lose" proposition. The organization would be "open to suit, i.e., by gays, if we attempt to exclude them, [and] by patients who might contract AIDS if we don't make every attempt to exclude gays, Haitians, and any other group associated with AIDS."

Cumming continued, the Red Cross was "liable to get more and more pressure to utilize those means." He predicted the pressure would come from CDC, which, he claimed, "needs a major epidemic to justify its existence."

But Cumming saw a way out from under CDC's thumb. The Red Cross could offer up its own strategy, one that would counter the effect of CDC's public criticism of blood bankers, and bolster Red Cross's image as responsible steward of the public health. The linchpin of that strategy: to discredit CDC. "To the extent the industry (ARC/CCBC/AABB) sticks together against CDC," Cumming wrote, "it will appear to some segments of the public at least that we have a self interest which is in conflict with the public interest, unless we can clearly demonstrate that CDC is wrong."

As the scenario now laid out, "within six to twelve months we won't have any choice but to use at least direct questioning and probably laboratory tests to 'attempt' to eliminate gay males."

Still, he had little faith in those measures. "How many men in Buffalo, New York are going to step forward out of their closet in front of their peers and admit they are 'queers'? Or even call in later to have their donation discarded?"

Despite the difference in positions over specific issues and solutions, the majority of Red Cross Blood Service officials surveyed seemed inclined to note the strong probability that AIDS was transmissible by blood and that the exposure could be minimized by a variety of methods aimed at excluding donors from high-risk groups.

On January 26, 1983, the same day he queried his officers, but before receiving their responses, Katz relayed to Red Cross blood centers headquarters' official position regarding AIDS screening. Blood regions should expand health history interviews to include specific questions concerning possible symptoms of or exposure to AIDS. But "there should be no direct questions concerning a donor's sexual preference, nor should a donor be asked to self-exclude on this basis." As for screening tests, "Routine laboratory tests to screen potential donors for AIDS are not recommended at this time."

On March 4, three months after CDC first warned the blood industry about AIDS, the Public Health Service promulgated "Inter Agency Recommendations" regarding the prevention of Acquired Immune Deficiency Syndrome in the blood supply. By then there were more than 400 AIDS deaths—out of a reported 1,100 cases. PHS recommended that sexual contact be avoided with persons known or suspected to have AIDS, and that high-risk groups "should refrain from donating plasma and/or blood." According to PHS, "Blood or blood products appear to be the vehicle responsible for the increased incidence of AIDS among hemophilia patients who require Factor VIII, a coagulating agent produced from pooling the blood of many donors."

As such, PHS advised blood and plasma collecting centers to suggest to high-risk individuals that they abstain from giving blood. Personnel responsible for donor screening should be retrained to recognize the telltale signs of AIDS, and standard operating procedures should include the quarantine and disposal of any product collected from a donor known or suspected to have AIDS.

PHS also recommended that studies be conducted by blood banks to "evaluate screening procedures for their effectiveness; those procedures should include specific laboratory tests."

But the agency fell short of advocating direct donor questioning about high-risk sexual activity. It did not recommend surrogate testing of donated blood. It also did not recommend screening the millions of units of blood already in stock. Over 1.5 million units had been collected between January and March of 1983 alone.

Among those who criticized PHS's weak position was the country's foremost clinical expert in AIDS. Dr. Marcus Conant, a professor at the University of California Medical Center at San Francisco and co-chair of the California State AIDS Leadership Committee, began observing, in the late 1970s, a peculiar skin condition in his dermatology practice. The condition mainly affected gay men. Within a few years Conant would treat 5,000 AIDS patients, both men and women. PHS's response to a major health care crisis was, Conant believed, "At best, nothing more than watered-down recommendations from the blood banking industry itself. At no time did the PHS and FDA bring into the review process individuals without ties to the blood industry who were expert in evaluation and treatment of patients with AIDS, or representatives from the hospital industry, American medicine, or, indeed, the general public who would be receiving the blood that was drawn from infected donors."

The cornerstone of the Red Cross's response to the PHS recommendations was to amend its regional flyer, *What You Should Know about Giving Blood.* Inserted on an 8 1/2-by-11-inch piece of paper folded into thirds were two paragraphs, less than 150 words, on AIDS. The Red Cross described this disease as "an illness of unknown cause . . . believed spread by intimate personal contact and possibly blood transfusions." There was no mention that it was fatal, only that "persons with AIDS have reduced defenses against disease and as a result may develop infections such as pneumonia or other serious illness."

The Red Cross reiterated, "At this time there is no laboratory test to detect blood that is capable of transmitting AIDS."

The Red Cross flyer was all that stood between AIDS and recipients of the Red Cross blood.

CHAPTER SIX

DOLLARS AND CENTS
1984

*[Washington D.C.] has found some positive donors whose
units have been transfused.*

Dr. Harold Lamberson
The American Red Cross
1984

In early May of 1983, a frequent donor in the San Francisco Bay area
entered Stanford University's blood bank, an affiliate of Stanford's
Medical Center. There he was given information about AIDS: its high
mortality rate, absence of clear-cut symptoms, and its potential transmissibility through blood. His blood was then drawn and subjected
to, among other routine tests, a T-cell blood test. The T-cell test was
an indicator of a severe immune deficiency that characterized AIDS
patients.

Because of an abnormality in his T-cell count, the donor was rejected by Stanford, which discarded his blood. His blood was accepted, however, at the Red Cross San Jose blood center and
subsequently transfused.

Like other Red Cross collection sites, San Jose was following headquarters policy: there was no surrogate blood testing and no direct
questioning concerning any donor's lifestyle.

About nine months later, the donor, a bisexual man, was dead of
AIDS.

Shortly after the first cases of AIDS were reported in 1981, it became apparent to Stanford Blood Bank director Dr. Edgar Engleman
that this disease was caused by an infectious agent that could be transmitted by blood.

In the spring of 1983, he had treated his first clear-cut cases of transfusion AIDS whose only risk factor had been their receipt of blood transfusions at Bay Area institutions within the past three years.

There was still no specific test to detect the AIDS virus, and the causal agent had not yet been found. But Engleman believed it ill advised to wait. He began aggressively exploring blood tests that could at least reduce the incidence of transmission through blood.

T-cells had long been of interest to Engleman. These were a class of white blood cells crucial to the body's ability to fight infection. In AIDS patients, suppresser cells which keep the immune system from running amok had been found to outnumber healthy "helper" T-cells. The AIDS patient's immune system thus was stripped and he or she became vulnerable to infections that a healthy person can easily thwart. T-cell abnormalities were, therefore, more indicative of the presence of an immune suppression by HIV than the presence of hepatitis core antibodies. In July 1983, Stanford became the first in the nation to screen donated blood with a surrogate blood test, in this case the T-cell test. T-cell testing met all the criteria for a surrogate test that the blood industry claimed to need. It was highly specific to AIDS, reliable, reproducible, and fast. While the test would probably not identify all AIDS carriers and would incorrectly identify a few individuals who were not carriers at all, Engleman nonetheless felt that the benefits of preventing some AIDS-contaminated blood from entering the blood supply outweighed those disadvantages.

Stanford was soon screening about 150 donors a day, in about two and a half hours. The cost of T-cell equipment was initially high, but the test added only between $10 and $12 per donor screening. To compensate, Stanford charged hospitals an additional 10 percent, raising the price of a unit of red cells, for example, from $60 to $66. Hospitals did not object, particularly as surgery candidates began choosing facilities supplied by Stanford blood; the perception was that blood from Edgar Engleman's lab was "safer."

In initiating surrogate testing, Engleman did not intend to set Stanford apart from, or embarrass, the blood banking community. Quite the contrary: he considered himself part of an establishment that had generally served the public well. But early on he had made a decision to exit the blood banking's political loop. Politics did not belong in medicine, but it still played an integral part in blood bankers' decisions. There was little, if any, resistance to industry policies from the agency that regulated blood, the FDA. Engleman characterized the FDA's Blood Products Advisory Committee as comprised largely of industry members. It was self-regulating and monolithic.

Engleman knew the Red Cross had been irate when Stanford had announced, in the 1970s, that it was going to open its own blood bank. Stanford had taken that step because Engleman had been unhappy with the Red Cross's ability to provide adequate blood to the medical center. Still, he was surprised at the hostility he encountered when he initiated the T-cell test. He had tried to convey the urgency of surrogate testing at the annual national meeting of the American Association of Blood Banks. Engleman's early findings had already confirmed reports from CDC that AIDS patients showed a reduced ratio of CD4 (helper) to CD8 (suppresser) T-cells, as did other likely carriers of the AIDS pathogen. He had submitted an abstract in which he described how T-cell testing was done, and he offered to help any blood bank get started.

But his abstract was rejected for presentation. Engleman later learned that transfusion AIDS was barely addressed on the meeting's agenda.

Shortly after Engleman began T-cell testing, the FDA received complaints that Stanford was using an unlicensed test, despite the fact that many of the tests blood bankers used were not licensed. Stanford's Office of the President also began receiving anonymous phone calls accusing Engleman of financial impropriety. The callers claimed he was "profiting" from the surrogate test. When the accusations persisted, Stanford was forced to investigate. No evidence whatsoever was found to implicate Engleman or anyone in the blood bank of any wrongdoing.

It was soon apparent that the "profiteers" from Stanford's blood testing policy were the blood recipients themselves. From July 1983 to June 1985, Stanford would handle a total of 33,831 blood donations. Of those donations, 586 donors, or 1.7 percent, tested for abnormal T-cell ratios. That blood was discarded, but Engleman retained rejected samples for future confirmatory testing should an AIDS-specific test became available.

The accuracy of the T-cell surrogate would be borne out when in March 1985 the AIDS specific test was put on the market. Using the new "ELISA" test, which could detect the virus that caused AIDS, Engleman retested those positive samples. The T-cell test he had employed nearly two years earlier had failed to detect only 0.2 percent of high-risk donors.

By preventing 586 infected donors from entering the blood pool between July 1983 and March 1985, Stanford spared as many as 33 patients from acquiring transfusion AIDS and potentially spreading it.

The Red Cross plasma division had already begun to feel the economic cost of failing to screen blood. In the spring, it had recalled two lots of Factor VIII concentrate when it learned that a donor to the pool had died of AIDS. Those lots contained nearly 5,600 vials of Factor VIII, which had been distributed to fifteen Red Cross blood service regions. Those vials would have treated 200 to 300 hemophiliacs for two to three months, or a single patient for eight years.

Hyland Therapeutics Labs, which fractionated plasma for the Red Cross, had also voluntarily recalled two lots of Factor IX: about 1,000 vials produced from a Red Cross contaminated pool. Another plasma company recalled 15 presumably AIDS-infected units.

The international market was losing confidence in U.S. blood. France had banned its importation. The United Kingdom was considering the same. Spain and Germany were discussing the effect such a ban would have on the availability of blood product in their country.

On December 15 and 16, 1983 the year-end Blood Products Advisory Committee meeting was held at the Lister Hill Auditorium on the campus of the National Institutes of Health. It was co-sponsored by the National Heart, Lung and Blood Institute and the Office of Biologics. Dr. William Miller was again acting chairman. Among the dozens of industry representatives listed as attending were Red Cross officials Alfred Katz, Joseph O'Malley and Roger Dodd.

By now, the CDC had identified twenty-nine AIDS patients who were not in the known high-risk groups. Their only risk had been receipt of blood during the past five years. At least one high-risk donor had been implicated in virtually every case. Fourteen of those patients were still alive. Could the deaths have been averted? At the BPAC meeting, several participants made strong cases for surrogate blood testing to cull out high-risk donors. Thomas Spira, chief of the CDC's Immunology Lab, presented staggering correlations between hepatitis core positive test results and AIDS. Among patients in the high-risk groups, the frequencies of positive individuals were homosexual males (88.1 percent) IV drug users (96.3 percent) and Haitians (80 percent.)

Prompted by recent plasma withdrawals resulting from a traceback to an AIDS donor, Red Cross contractor Hyland Labs had conducted a study of surrogate testing. Test results of plasma samples taken from 1,156 donors showed that 16 percent would have been rejected had the surrogate test been used to screen those units.

Dr. Johanna Pindyck of the New York Blood Center urged BPAC to consider recommendations for core testing in light of its implications for the voluntary sector. "If [anti HBc testing] is good to do," she said, "then it is good to do for all blood donations. . . . One would have to consider very seriously whether one could release any product [for transfusion] that couldn't be put into a pool for a hemophilia population."

Irwin Memorial Blood Bank's Dr. Herbert Perkins argued that the surrogate tests eliminated too many donors and could threaten the adequacy of the blood supply. The high proportion of positives from known gays suggested that the test was not distinguishing gays who may be carriers of AIDS from those who were not. Stanford's Dr. Edgar Engleman countered with his T-cell specific findings. As for cost, one hospitalization of an AIDS patient would, Engleman noted, justify the cost of the tests and equipment.

The data on surrogate testing was enough to convince FDA blood chief Dennis Donohue that plasma should be tested and he said so at the meeting. Plasma makers did not welcome the FDA's intrusion on their largely self-regulated industry. On the evening of December 15, several of the leading clotting factor manufacturers met. By the end of the night they had come up with a counter-proposal.

After the general BPAC meeting the following day, the manufacturers told Donohue that they had formed a task force to study anticore testing. In an internal memo, a Cutter Labs director reported: "The general thrust of the task force is to provide a delaying tactic for the implementation of further testing. . . . Although Donohue was not completely satisfied by the task force approach, he agreed to it." The task force included Dr. Peter Page of the Red Cross. Months later, it would conclude that surrogate testing was not warranted.

The Red Cross's Fred Katz had apparently taken to heart presentations made at the BPAC meeting. On December 20, the director of Red Cross Blood Services issued a priority directive to his regions. He informed them that the hepatitis B core antibody was among the many tests the BPAC was considering. "One report indicated that anti-HBc was found in 80 percent or more of AIDS patients or persons considered at risk for developing AIDS." Katz did not advise any changes in blood or donor screening policy. But he issued a series of confidential staff assignments at headquarters. He requested that Sandler, Cumming and other key officers "critically re-evaluate the possibility of the introduction of anti HBc as a donor screening test."

Fred Katz wanted a cost benefit analysis and information on surrogate test manufacturers' capabilities.

The new year began on an alarming note for the Red Cross. In early January of 1984, headquarters learned the results of surrogate blood test trials of its donors in various cities, including Boston, Philadelphia, Los Angeles, Cleveland, Washington, and Buffalo. On January 10, Roger Dodd sent a memo to Fred Katz, via Gerald Sandler, indicating that Red Cross donors who were at high risk for AIDS, were *still giving blood*. Of 1,650 donors tested in Los Angeles alone, nearly 7 percent were hepatitis core positive. Five percent of a sample of 335 donors in several other cities including Washington, D.C. were also core positive. Of a total of nearly 40,000 randomly tested Red Cross donors, about 3 percent were core positive.

The Red Cross now had a national profile of its donors. That data indicated that self deferral by AIDS high risk groups was not working.

In his memo to Fred Katz concerning these test results, Roger Dodd pointed out, "More than eighty percent of AIDS patients and male homosexuals judged to be at high risk of developing AIDS are reactive for HBc." Should the Red Cross initiate surrogate testing, Dodd predicted, "The repeat donor population would be depleted of reactive donors."

At the heels of the Dodd memo, Katz received a sobering message from Sandler. It seemed he was no longer willing to dismiss surrogate testing.

"Anti HBc negative blood," Sandler told Katz, "is safer."

In light of the evidence the Red Cross now had that high-risk, core positive donors were giving blood, surrogate testing could ensure that those who did not self defer were not accepted into the blood registry.

At $5 per test, the cost to screen out high-risk donors would be about $60 million a year. Sandler told Katz that this outlay was "justifiable in light of projected benefits."

Despite certain public relations glitches ("adding to the confusion and increasing anxiety"), Sandler told Katz, "Testing for anti HBc is a reasonable, indirect, if not direct, approach to predicting AIDS exposure."

By early 1984, blood bankers could not agree on specific preventive measures, but they did agree that AIDS was blood borne. In mid-February, CDC met with industry members to discuss what studies needed to be done. As Dr. Joe Bove, head of the Transfusion Transmitted Diseases Committee, conveyed to his members, including the Red Cross, "There was a general agreement that studies to determine whether AIDS is transmitted by blood have relatively low priority, since nearly everyone agrees it probably is."

If AIDS were, as industry leaders seemed to concur, blood borne, then why the reluctance to surrogate test? A March 20, 1984 internal memo from the Red Cross's Paul Cumming offered some insight into organization's priorities.

Cumming had designed a cost matrix weighing the financial considerations of surrogate testing versus the benefits. He determined that "Objectively it is difficult to make a case for adoption of AIDS marker testing." The cost for testing in all Red Cross blood regions would range, Cumming estimated, from $15 million to $67 million. "If we assume that each averted AIDS case has the value of $1 million, then to justify use of one of the tests would require an expected reduction in tfx [transfusion-associated]-AIDS from ARC blood of 15 to 67 cases."

But a life value of $1 million per AIDS-infected transfusion patient was, Cumming thought, high. "Since tfx-AIDS patients have an average 50 years of age, average earnings per worker are approximately $20,000 per annum, and treatment for AIDS victims has averaged about $80,000, the likely value of an averted tfx-AIDS case is about $500,000. This lower benefit would indicate a need to prevent 30 to 134 tfx-AIDS cases from ARC to justify use of a marker test exclusively on economic considerations. In addition, these averted cases would have to be over and above the number of cases prevented by currently implemented screening measures."

Cumming went on to explain, "To economically justify anti HBc testing in all Blood Service regions, we would need to demonstrate an anticipated rate of tfx-AIDS (not prevented by screening measures) of 1.75 cases per week, assuming an 88 percent effectiveness rate of the test." That rate, he noted, was "considerably above prior and current rates."

Cumming predicted at most a *possible* 50 cases per year of AIDS avoided" [emphasis in original]. To compensate 50 individuals who might be infected by HIV-contaminated blood could cost Red Cross, at $500,000 per victim, about $25 million, far less than the high-end $67 million to screen HIV from the blood supply.

He did not mention that the high-end cost of $67 million represented about 6.5 percent of Red Cross Blood Services processing revenue for 1984 alone.

Cumming concluded that "Implementation of any AIDS marker test will be extremely expensive. Given the fact that tfx-AIDS is still a hypothesis, that there has been no effective measurement of the success of the screening procedures which have already been implemented, and that cost justification of testing would rest on a considerably higher incidence of tfx-AIDS than is currently being observed."

The number of cases of transfusion AIDS that could be prevented by surrogate testing did not justify the expense. It appeared it would be cheaper to pay off infected blood recipients, should they pursue legal action, than to clean up the Red Cross blood supply.

There were, however, other factors to consider; these were in the marketing and public welfare areas. "Namely, plasma industry projected adoption of such a test is a rather obvious marketing initiative which will serve to increase pressure on us. Furthermore, Red Cross decision-making criteria are complicated by considerations or ethics and public welfare as distinct from competitive response."

It was not until March 1984 that the San Jose blood region of the American Red Cross learned that it had, a year earlier, accepted a confirmed AIDS infected donor. Dr. Pearl Toy, director of the Central California Region, also learned that the donor, who had since died, had been accepted at the Peninsula Blood Bank as well. Units donated to San Jose and Peninsula had long been transfused. This same donor had been rejected by Stanford University Blood Bank which had used the T-cell surrogate blood test.

As a result of this incident, Toy had re-examined the surrogate test issue, specifically the effectiveness of hepatitis anticore. She was surprised at its sensitivity. A random sampling of "neighborhood gay controls" showed 77 percent were anticore positive, as were 91 percent of gays at VD clinics. This data, coupled with the economic pressure in the Bay area to surrogate test, convinced Pearl Toy that San Jose had to depart from headquarters' policy.

On March 29, Toy sent a letter to Gerald Sandler informing him of the situation and "evidence that active homosexuals in the Bay area are still donating blood." One sexually active gay donor, for instance, did not self defer. He did not consider himself at high risk for AIDS. "This way of thinking unfortunately is not unique among local active homosexual men," Toy told Sandler.

Her Medical Advisory Committee had decided to initiate anticore.

A few weeks later, Dr. Lauren O'Brien, San Jose's acting medical director, wrote Katz of their plan to implement core screening as early as June 1. O'Brien assured Katz that San Jose would be diplomatic in informing any donors of positive test results: "No mention of anti HBc as a marker for those in a high-risk group for AIDS will be made."

San Jose intended to add a surcharge of $4 to each blood product it sold in order to cover the cost of testing and the loss of some good blood. It would also make sure that each donor read and understood the pamphlet *What You Should Know about Giving Blood.* Intake personnel were told, "If there is any doubt in your mind, repeat the pertinent questions about symptoms, contacts, etc."

When San Jose announced its intent to surrogate test, headquarters knew it had a problem. That rebel act could set a precedent among other regions, endangering the industry's agreed-upon "standard of care," which exempted the Red Cross from costly test initiatives. Furthermore, San Jose's policy could create public confusion, a rift in the perception of a united Red Cross. The blood banker had too publicly criticized surrogate testing to tolerate this sort of mutiny.

The Red Cross had previously been successful in preventing other blood banks from straying from the industry's standard practices. That meant no direct donor questioning, and no surrogate blood tests. In 1983, for example, the organization prevented the Blood Bank at Charity Hospital in New Orleans, a collection and transfusion service for Louisiana State University School of Medicine and Tulane University School of Medicine, from implementing surrogate testing. The Charity Hospital blood bank was headed by Dr. David DeJongh. DeJongh had vigorously recommended to his board the need for surrogate tests. He told them that it was "widely known that routine screening for core antibody (anti HBc) would reduce the risk for both hepatitis B virus and non A–non B hepatitis."

DeJongh would not be allowed to conduct surrogate blood tests. In an affidavit he submitted in a 1987 transfusion-AIDS lawsuit against the Red Cross (later presented at a Congressional subcommittee hearing) DeJongh wrote, "We were unable to institute the test at our hospital because the committees that were designed to make these determinations felt pressure, particularly from the blood industry, including the American Red Cross. The pressure that was asserted was designed to keep blood banks from straying from the course set by the blood industry, including the Red Cross, that course being to avoid the use of the core antibody test."

Fred Katz dispatched Roger Dodd, assistant director of the Transmissible Diseases and Immunology Lab, to try to dissuade San Jose from initiating surrogate testing. Dodd was armed with news of an AIDS specific blood test which was expected to hit the market in November 1984.

At an April 23, 1984 press conference, Secretary of Health and Human Services Margaret Heckler announced that the infectious agent for AIDS had been found. AIDS, it seemed, was a retrovirus, a variant of an infectious HTLV agent implicated in a type of human cancer. Heckler told the public and the press, "We now have a blood test for AIDS which we hope can be widely available within about six months."

That test would identify AIDS with 100-percent certainty. But to many industry experts, the announcement was premature. Even the more optimistic did not expect a viable test within a six-month window.

Robert Gallo, chief of the National Cancer Institute's Lab, Tumor Cell Biology, was credited with the discovery.

Heckler's optimism aside, West Coast blood banks, including Irwin Memorial and the Blood Bank of the Alameda–Contra Costa Medical Association, decided to adopt surrogate testing. Their test of choice was the very one CDC's Don Francis had urged blood banks adopt two years earlier: hepatitis anticore.

"Heckler's announcement took the heat off the Red Cross," Don Francis later explained. "It gave them another year to rationalize doing nothing."

Heckler also provided the Red Cross with the ammunition it needed to attempt to quash rebellion among centers like San Jose. In a deposition Roger Dodd gave in a later transfusion-AIDS case brought against the Red Cross, he recalled his mission to San Jose. "I believed and others at headquarters believed that we would have access to test for antibodies to HTLV-III, and we felt that it was a very good opportunity to put the test which clearly was going to be the test for AIDS into a protocol. Since San Jose was adamant about initiating an additional test anyway, it seemed reasonable to suggest to them that they might wait to consider HTLV-III antibody testing. So at that level, I certainly suggested to them they might want to consider that as an alternate approach."

When San Jose opted not to wait, Fred Katz reminded administrator Pearl Toy, "American Red Cross Blood Services recommends that all regional Blood Services do not perform nonspecific tests for AIDS, since there is no evidence that such testing will reduce the number of cases of transfusion-associated AIDS." Still, he had to acknowledge that the Central California region had been placed in a sensitive competitive position.

Katz's solution to San Jose's "departure from Blood Services recommended policy" was to designate it as a test site. He proposed to Toy that she introduce anti HBc testing as a "six-month study" to evaluate the impact of this test on her blood donor program. San Jose was deemed Red Cross's "experiment" in surrogate screening, presumably to supply headquarters with usable data. So was the Red Cross's Pennsylvania New Jersey Region (Penn-Jersey), the other insubordinate center, which chose to directly question donors.

San Jose would learn what diligent blood collectors who followed Edgar Engleman's lead had: that high-risk donors were not self-deferring, and that surrogate tests screened out high-risk donors.

San Jose was not the only region bearing ominous news to headquarters.

The AIDS epidemic and HIV testing were among the subjects discussed at a May 23 meeting of the Red Cross's Medical Advisory Committee. Dr. Harold Lamberson, medical director of the Syracuse, New York blood region, told the group that there appeared to be some leveling off of reported AIDS in "hot spots" like New York and San Francisco. However, he explained, it was difficult to interpret the rate at which the disease was spreading because of its long incubation period. Lamberson predicted, "Since the disease has been recognized for only two years, the number of transfusion-related cases will most likely increase."

Lamberson was interrupted in his AIDS discourse by committee participant Dr. Nosanchuk. As the meeting minutes indicated, "Dr. Nosanchuk asked why such a big deal is being made out of AIDS." Similar resources were not, he pointed out, allocated to non A-non B hepatitis, which was a significant problem.

His colleague Dr. Kagan replied that there was a difference between hepatitis and AIDS. "Non A-non B may lead to morbidity in a small number of patients," Kagan said. "But AIDS so far has been fatal in all."

The discussion moved on to the AIDS specific test, also known as the ELISA test. Requests were being submitted to FDA for early access to the tests. Nosanchuk questioned its effectiveness in non laboratory settings.

Lamberson then dropped the bombshell. "The Red Cross has access to that [HTLV-III] test," he said. "They have tested fifteen hundred samples from the Washington, D.C. center. They have, in fact, found some positive donors whose units have been transfused."

The shocking news that HIV-confirmed positive donors were giving blood apparently raised only one question: what were the ethical issues of informing recipients and donors that they had AIDS?

"There needs to be good recording, in the event a cure is found for this disease," Kagan said, "so transfused individuals and donors can then be appropriately followed up for treatment."

Discussion then proceeded to non-AIDS related matters.

The fact that Red Cross had recent evidence that *HIV test positive* donors had given blood in D.C. and that blood had been transfused appeared to have created barely a ripple of interest at the meeting.

Less than two months later, on July 2, 1984, Hailey, Heather and Holly Michaels were transfused with drops of HIV-infected blood from that Washington D.C. center. A month later, Roland Ray was similarly infected with AIDS.

CHAPTER SEVEN

THE PUBLIC BE DAMNED

1985–1989

Gifts of money. Of time. Of blood. Freely given. So that others will benefit. So that others will find hope.

1989 Annual Report
The American Red Cross

To allay public fears, the Department of Health and Human Services had gone way out on a limb. It promised the country an AIDS test by November 1984, only six months after it announced the discovery of the HIV virus. The Reagan administration, which had been largely indifferent to the AIDS crisis, undoubtedly recognized a showcase opportunity for the President's second-term bid.

The competition to win FDA's first license, and hence the lion's share of a $70 million domestic ($180 million worldwide) market, was fierce. About 23 million tests were going to be needed by the 2,300 blood banks and plasma centers nationwide. The Red Cross alone would require an estimated 6 million kits a year. In the running were Abbott Laboratories, the $5 billion blood-testing equipment company, which had already cornered the market for hepatitis B test kits; Electro Nucleonics; and three joint ventures that partnered Litton Bionetics with Johnson & Johnson, Genetech with Baxter Travenol, and Biotech Research Labs with Du Pont, and Genetic Systems, a small company in Seattle.

By year end, there was still no AIDS test on the market. There were, instead, major technical problems. In comparative studies conducted by the Public Health Service and in confirming trials by manufacturers, the ability of the kits to screen blood accurately for the virus that caused AIDS varied widely. Abbott's tests were registering false positives as well as false negatives. Healthy donors might be diagnosed as HIV positive and rejected while HIV-infected donors could be cleared into the donation pool.

Compounding these operational glitches were sensitive political issues involving potential stigmatization of HIV-positive individuals. The notion of giving the test free of charge and making blood centers the sole testing sites also raised concerns. High-risk groups could attempt to give blood to obtain a free AIDS test. Virus-infected blood could potentially slip through. Taking steps to rid the blood supply of HIV might actually increase risks of contamination.

Dr. Peter Page of the Red Cross expressed concern about the government's urgency to market the AIDS test. He told *Nature* magazine in December 1984, "We're being rushed so much by Margaret Heckler [Secretary of Health and Human Services] that we don't have time to resolve [the problems]." Page questioned the need for any AIDS test. Self-deferral among high-risk groups was, he claimed, highly effective at Red Cross centers where voluntary abstention had significantly improved the safety of the blood supply. Page saw no compelling reason for a blood test that would "add a relatively small increment of safety."

Purchasing and implementing the AIDS tests could cost the Red Cross about $20 million a year. The cost would be about two dollars per test.

Still, the Red Cross began clinical tests of several kits, including those developed by Abbott Labs and Genetic Systems. Problems notwithstanding, the Red Cross chose Abbott. When Abbott became the first company to win FDA approval in March 1985, it immediately laid claim to about sixty percent of the market.

The ELISA (enzyme-linked immunosorbent assay), as the AIDS test was called, was relatively simple. A small amount of blood taken from a donor was mixed with an isolated, safe sample of the HIV virus. If an antibody were present it would adhere to particles of the virus, called antigens (surface proteins). When a chemical reagent was introduced, the antigens would change to green, yellow, or blue. The test could not detect the HTLV-III virus per se, only the presence of antibodies to fight it. It could not determine whether an individual had AIDS, only whether he or she had developed antibodies through exposure to HIV.

While the process was fairly standard, the species of the virus, or the "clinical isolate," was not. With the exception of Genetic Systems,

Abbott and other licensed test manufacturers used "H9" cells obtained from Robert Gallo's lab. Genetic Systems used the lymphadenopathy associated virus (LAV) marketed through Pasteur Diagnostics. The LAV virus known in the United States as the HIV virus had been isolated in 1983 at the Pasteur Institute in France. Pasteur Diagnostics had the right to sell various products derived from the institute's research. Citing its discovery of LAV, the Pasteur Institute was challenging Gallo's claim to virus isolation.

When Abbott began production of its kits, its false readings had not been resolved. The St. Paul region of the Red Cross was among the first to become aware of the defects. In March 1985, St. Paul had begun routinely using the AIDS test as part of its blood screening. In December it undertook a comparative study of kits made by Abbott, Du Pont Labs, and Genetic Systems. St. Paul found that Genetic Systems outperformed the Abbott test, which tallied up over 800 inaccurate readings. The Genetic Systems test was, St. Paul concluded, "consistent with our philosophy of using the best product available to ensure the safety of blood, while also employing the test that allows us to fully use as many donations as possible and thereby to minimize costs."

A Canadian government study of test kits also found, "Abbott kits consistently failed to correctly identify serum that contained *only* the antibody to P24 [an antigen—that is, a protein component of HIV]." The presence of P24 was an early sign of HIV infection. Abbott did not screen for P24; Genetic Systems did.

Tests conducted by other Red Cross centers during the year found that Abbott's error rate for false readings was over seventy percent. By the summer of 1985, the Red Cross learned that at least one recipient of its blood, which had been screened by Abbott, had contracted transfusion AIDS.

Abbott assured the Red Cross it would make necessary improvements. By year end there were still no significant changes.

Two months later, in February 1986, a Red Cross task force compared several AIDS test kits. Again, Genetic Systems proved superior to Abbott. Among Abbott's problems: nonrepeatable results, leaky vials, sensitivity variances, and "low positive control." In May 1986 alone, Abbott had to replace its kits in Detroit; Roanoke, Virginia; Johnson City, Tennessee; Durham, Charlotte, and Winston-Salem, North Carolina; Galesburg, Illinois; Syracuse, New York; Tucson, Arizona; and Tulsa, Oklahoma. About 7,500 tests had to be replaced in Durham and 12,000 in Charlotte, North Carolina.

Abbott sent a mailgram the following month to the Syracuse Red Cross announcing FDA approval of its "new formulation for improved HTLV-III antibody reagents." That test promised "enhanced specificity." There were, however, some skeptics about the test's performance. Dr. Harold Lamberson, Red Cross Blood Services director in Syracuse, scribbled a note to a colleague on that mailgram: "I'm not sure I believe this."

The Red Cross also learned the results of a two-year National Institutes of Health study which tracked nearly 5,000 homosexual and bisexual men in Baltimore, Chicago, Los Angeles, and Pittsburgh. NIH epidemiologist Dr. Alfred J. Saah had been testing blood samples from that group since 1984 at six-month intervals. He and his researchers discovered that the same blood was testing antibody negative with some kits and antibody positive with others. At an NIH Consensus Conference, Saah told blood bankers, including Red Cross representatives, that of the 30 samples testing early-stage core positive, Abbott detected 43 percent, Genetic Systems, 83 percent. Abbott had missed 17 of the samples; Genetic Systems, only 5. Electro Nucleonics, which screened blood for the military, missed 26 of the 30.

Dr. Peter Tomasulo, director of the Red Cross's South Florida regional Blood Services, was impressed by Dr. Saah's presentation. He conveyed his concerns about the Red Cross's continued use of the Abbott test to a colleague at the Red Cross Omaha blood region. "I developed the strong impression," Tomasulo wrote, "that our blood center should start using Genetic Systems or Du Pont to detect HTLV-III antibody. It looks like those assays detected the antibody to the P24 antigen better than the Abbott assay and it looks like P24 reliably correlates with early HTLV-III infection. I'm more concerned that the South Florida region should consider a switch. When I broaden my concerns for the whole Red Cross system, my conviction is even stronger."

Each month, South Florida transfused more than 500,000 red cells and other blood components. Citing a donor who had tested HIV negative on the Abbott test but was, in fact, positive, Tomasulo told his Omaha colleague, "We know we have a better chance of detecting such an individual by using the Genetic Systems assay. Delaying the switch even one month may be wrong. If one person in South Florida develops AIDS from a seronegative blood donor after July 30, 1986 which was processed by Abbott, I will wonder if I did everything I could have done."

Still, the Red Cross renewed its contract with Abbott for another year. It gave the manufacturer eighty-five percent of its market.

At a Red Cross Center Directors Council meeting in San Francisco on November 1, 1986, Abbott's report on the "excellent" performance of its "tuned" kits was discussed. As reflected in the meeting minutes, one Red Cross blood official suggested that only a "limited amount of faith could be put in this report." Syracuse's Director Dr. Lamberson had conducted his own comparative study of Abbott, Genetic Systems, and Du Pont tests. He told Red Cross executives Drs. Sandler, Lew Barker, Fred Katz, Leon Hoyer, Victor Schmitt, and J. B. Schorr that Abbott had failed to detect the "1" case among "23" suspect cases which had progressed to full-blown AIDS.

Lamberson wrote, "A screening test such as Du Pont or Genetic Systems [which] readily identified samples with antibody to HIV core proteins alone is essential for use in blood banks."

Sandler was worried about the "several unexplained delays" in Abbott's submitting its "new" kits for FDA approval. Sandler advised that the Red Cross use a more sensitive test. As reflected in the minutes, vice president Barker offered the perspective that no blood center would likely be held negligent for using an FDA approved procedure, even if other procedures were more sensitive.

By the end of 1986, Abbott still had not improved its tests. On December 22, Red Cross Council members, including Peter Tomasulo, Sandler, and Lamberson, conferred by phone. They discussed several Red Cross regions' "strong desire" to switch from Abbott to another manufacturer. But the Council decided that Abbott should be given another chance.

In mid-January 1987, almost two years after the Red Cross had learned of Abbott's test kit defects, the manufacturer received FDA approval for its upgraded test kits. In the interim misdiagnosis through faulty readings had resulted in tragedies. An initial review by CDC in February 1988 found that thirteen people who had received blood from donors who had tested negative by Abbott had contracted transfusion AIDS; twelve of those blood recipients had no other risk factor than blood transfusion. Among those victims were twin sisters transfused in 1986.

In a medical paper written by the CDC's AIDS Program, the authors concluded, "The number of persons who have become infected with HIV after receiving [apparently] seronegative blood from infected donors is probably several times larger than the thirteen reported here. Even an approximate number was difficult to determine since the estimated 3 to 4 million recipients of blood annually are not routinely tested subsequently for HIV antibody."

In 1987 as the Abbott issue was being resolved, the Red Cross faced its first significant legal challenge, the Kozup transfusion-AIDS lawsuit.

Matthew Kozup was born by cesarean section on January 9, 1983. He weighed barely three pounds. During his stay at Georgetown Hospital, he received twenty transfusions of minute quantities of blood. One of the donors had AIDS. At least five other premature infants had also been transfused with HIV-contaminated blood at Georgetown, one of sixty hospitals in the D.C. area served by the Red Cross.

Matthew spent most of his short life in hospitals. He never weighed more than twenty pounds. His body was scarred with puncture marks made by needles. The HIV virus lowered his resistance to a range of diseases, and he was forced to live in isolation, much of the time in pain. His medical bills exceeded $350,000.

On the day he turned three and a half years old, Matthew died of AIDS. His parents claimed in their negligence lawsuit that the Red Cross and Georgetown Hospital had known about AIDS since 1979. As such, the blood supplier and hospital should have informed the Kozups about the risks of blood transfusions and obtained their informed consent.

Matthew Kozup v. the American Red Cross hinged on the critical issue of timing: exactly when did the Red Cross know HIV was transmitted by blood? Did the Red Cross have this knowledge prior to Matthew's blood transfusions?

The Red Cross was prepared to fight back aggressively with claims of its own ignorance. It immediately moved for summary judgment—dismissal for lack of merit. The Red Cross told the court that in early 1983 it had not yet known that the AIDS virus was transmissible by blood. Therefore, it had not been obligated to inform the Kozups of the potential risk of blood-borne AIDS. Furthermore, there was no AIDS test available until March 1985. As a result, it had not breached its duty to provide adequate blood from safe donors, had not failed to screen high-risk donors, and had not erred in failing to conduct tests to eliminate AIDS in the blood supply.

The Red Cross likened Matthew's transfusion of AIDS to a natural disaster: "As often happens with disasters . . . they can occur without anyone to blame."

In making its decision to grant summary judgment, the United

States District Court for the District of Columbia relied almost exclusively on exhibits supplied by the Red Cross. Consequently, the court ruled, "No responsible jury could find that the possibility of contracting AIDS from a blood transfusion was a material risk at the time Matthew Kozup received his three transfusions. A risk of one in 3.5 million [based on the one reported transfusion AIDS case of the 20-month-old infant in San Francisco in 1982, versus 3.5 million blood donations annually], cannot be said to be material to a reasonable patient."

The court also decided in favor of the Red Cross on the product warranty and strict liability claim. It was, the judge ruled, "unnatural to force a blood transfusion into the ordinary commercial sales mold." The sale of blood was not considered a commercial transaction, even though the Red Cross had accepted money in exchange.

The Matthew Kozup lawsuit was a weak case. As such it made bad law. While in theory, the federal court ruling had no legal bearing on future state court decisions, in practice, its broad language vindicated the Red Cross from accountability in 1983. It had set a dangerous precedent. By refusing to allow the case to go to trial, the court told transfusion-AIDS victims that they had no factual basis on which to sue.

Other victims died before knowing they had been contaminated. Many claims were barred by the statute of limitations governing the time frame during which a claim could be filed. The two main issues regarding the statute of limitations for transfusion AIDS cases were: Must the victim bring his claim from the date he was infected, or when he showed symptoms of the disease or when he learned he was HIV positive? Or could he bring suit from the time he first learned that his illness was related to the blood bank's negligence? Was the victim subject to the medical malpractice or the ordinary negligence statutes of limitations? There was little consistency in state court rulings on these questions.

Blood banks were also protected by "blood shield" laws which made it virtually impossible to bring product liability or breach of warranty claims against the blood industry. States which had enacted such legislation had conferred immunity to blood providers by terming blood a "service," not a "product." Victims could not sue blood banks as they would a product manufacturer for strict liability, breach of warranty. The "defective product" claim would not hold.

Most cases hinged on proving negligence in the manner of "battery," the failure of blood banks to obtain consent for the transfusion procedure; to adequately screen high-risk donors; and to use surrogate tests as an early marker of AIDS risks. The most significant barrier to proving negligence was the industry's "standard of care" defense. Standard of care, the accepted customs and practices of an industry at a given time.

Early in 1983, the Red Cross, the American Association of Blood Banks, and the Council of Community Blood Banks had anticipated their legal liability for distributing a potentially dangerous product. With some foresight, their Joint Policy Statements in 1983 and 1984 did not require direct questioning of donors' sexual lifestyles. Nor did they require surrogate testing. In effect, those statements became the blood industry's standard of care, its insurance policy against future liability.

Suing the Red Cross posed particular problems. The organization was protected not only by law and industry policy, but by its unique "quasi-governmental" status. The American Red Cross charter stated that it had "the power to sue and be sued in courts of law and equity, State or Federal, within the jurisdiction of the United States." But as an "instrumentality of the United States," the Red Cross claimed it was protected by "sovereign immunity" from jury verdicts and paying monetary damages.

Another advantage of the Red Cross's status was its "discretionary" privilege. Discretionary function as applied to government agencies was intended to leave legislative and administrative policy decisions to experts who presumably had the greater public interest in mind. The Red Cross could call upon that privilege to circumvent accountability.

As a routine practice, Red Cross requested "protective orders" in transfusion-AIDS court cases. Such orders, which sealed documents from public view, were often requested by corporations facing negligence suits who feared exposure of "trade secrets." The party claiming the need for a protective order must prove to the court that injury would result from certain disclosures. The Red Cross argued that disclosure of its sensitive internal communications would confuse the public about the highly complex scientific, technical, and emotional nature of the AIDS issue. As an advocate of the public's peace of mind, the Red Cross did not wish to create undue anxiety over events that had occurred in the past. Such doubts could, it told the courts, result in decreased public confidence and decreased donations, which in turn would jeopardize the adequacy of the nation's blood supply.

In addition, the Red Cross claimed that protective orders would ease and expedite the process of discovery, thus further serving the public.

With rare exceptions, judges granted the Red Cross's requests for sweeping protective orders. In this manner thousands of Red Cross documents were sealed from the public, press, and plaintiff attorneys bringing suit on behalf of their clients.

Plaintiffs' counsel were thus limited in their ability to develop evidence because they could not coordinate efforts with other plaintiffs' counsel. Bound by court order, attorneys like Mike Feldman and Chris Tisi had to essentially reinvent the wheel. They could not share Red Cross documents with other plaintiff firms. They could not seek advice from those who had brought the Red Cross to court. Each lawsuit had to be constructed from ground zero.

Essentially, a legal "bubble" had been created around the Red Cross.

In the Andrea Wilson case, Feldman and Tisi believed that donor and blood screening could have spared the girl's life. The civil wrongful death lawsuit, charged that "The Red Cross procured and/or utilized contaminated blood and/or blood products that were ultimately given to the decedent without reasonably utilizing methods available to screen out blood donated by members of the high-risk groups." The Red Cross did not advise Mrs. Wilson that the blood or blood products could have been contaminated with the AIDS virus, or that the blood had been obtained in the absence of reasonably developed and implemented donor screening procedures.

The suit also charged the Red Cross did not provide Mrs. Wilson with alternatives to, or advise her of the risks of blood transfusions. Alternatives included informing recipients of directed donations, whereby a patient could ask family or friends to contribute blood prior to surgery.

To score a victory, Feldman and Tisi knew they had to build a fortress. If they assumed a defensive position, if they sat back while the Red Cross and its counsel, Arnold & Porter, attacked, they would be buried. The two plaintiff attorneys began the laborious process of learning about transfusion AIDS. They hired a scientist to teach them the basics of blood banking, wrangled with protective orders to obtain documents, took depositions, and began identifying expert witnesses. Finding expert witnesses willing to testify against the Red Cross was difficult. As members of a closed clique dominated by the Red Cross, most blood bankers had been affiliated with the organization at some point in their careers. Robert Jenner, a Maryland plaintiff attorney and author of the legal tome *Transfusion-Associated AIDS*, observed, "Expert witnesses for victims had to be either a renegade or outside the industry." Yet, if they had been excluded from the blood banking club, the Red Cross challenged their qualifications, often successfully. If they were federal employees, like Don Francis from CDC, they were precluded by government policy from testifying.

There was, however, one renegade who was able and willing to testify. After placing dozens of phone calls to the Stanford University Blood Bank, Mike Feldman reached Edgar Engleman. Dr. Engleman said he was only interested in working with attorneys who were committed to exposing the truth about blood bank negligence. Engleman agreed to be an expert witness in the Wilson case, should it proceed to trial.

Meanwhile, Tisi thought he had scored a coup. He had learned that a former high-level Red Cross official was willing to testify against the organization. That official told Tisi that he had considerable ammunition in the form of documents and that he was willing to be deposed. As Tisi later recalled, "He told me he had 'boxes of material from the Red Cross, information that would blow them out of the water.' Those were his exact words, I remember that clearly."

However, when the former executive arrived for his deposition, he was flanked by Red Cross lawyers. He denied ever having had such a conversation with Chris Tisi.

While the Red Cross was successfully convincing the courts that any alleged negligence had occurred in the past, its more recent practices were questionable. Shortly after Feldman and Tisi filed the Wilson complaint, FDA released the findings of its 1988 inspections of Red Cross blood regions. A total of over 2,500 units of blood not suitable for use had been released by the Red Cross and, in many cases, transfused. Much of that blood had tested HIV reactive.

One of the worst offenders was Red Cross's flagship collection center in Washington, D.C. The D.C. center was in longstanding violation of federal blood safety laws. There were significant delays in its implementing the federally mandated "Look-Back" program, which required blood banks to promptly inform transfusion-AIDS victims and infected donors. A thorough investigation of AIDS cases from as far back as 1984 had still not been undertaken. Fewer than half a dozen of the 235 transfusion-AIDS victims from the D.C. center had been contacted: sixteen cases had occurred *after* HIV testing had begun in March 1985. Most of the 300 donors who had tested HIV reactive had also not been informed. Donor history files were so haphazard that FDA inspectors were unable to locate 4,500 records essential in tracing HIV-reactive donors and blood recipients.

Other regions were in equally dangerous disarray. Toledo, Ohio; Waco, Texas; Portland, Oregon; Mobile, Alabama; Little Rock, Arkansas; Albany, New York; Great Falls, Montana were among centers nationwide which were shipping out questionable blood for further manufacture or transfusion. In Nashville, test records of at least 8,735 units of whole blood drawn during March 1986 were missing, lost, or otherwise unavailable for inspection, including records of blood typing and testing for hepatitis, syphilis, and HIV. Approximately 18,000 blood components had been manufactured from those units. Throughout 1987, the Nashville center failed to adequately identify, quarantine, and incinerate units collected from donors testing reactive for HIV and hepatitis. The result: those units were distributed to hospitals and other blood centers for transfusion.

In Rochester, New York, failures in the donor deferral process in 1985 and 1986 resulted in the subsequent distribution of HIV-reactive units. In Albany, New York, 7 donors who had tested HIV reactive as early as 1985 still had not been deferred. In Norfolk, Virginia, 399 units obtained from donors with fluctuating HIV test results were distributed. In Cleveland, Ohio, "quarantined" blood was shipped to hospitals, plasma fractionators, and other Red Cross Blood Service regions.

At the Huntington, West Virginia Red Cross, blood acquired from 34 HIV-reactive donors who were deferred en masse on April 30, 1987, had been distributed.

Since 1985, the Farmington, Connecticut center had been accepting donors who were testing reactive for HIV. FDA would later learn that 255 HIV-reactive units had been released between April 1985 and August 1990 because the staff did not update the donor deferral files.

In Bethesda, Maryland a donor who had tested HIV reactive in 1988 would donate 12 more times; 11 of those donations were transfused into patients.

One of the largest recalls took place in Charlotte, North Carolina. There about 1,600 blood products that had tested reactive for HIV or hepatitis had been released. Los Angeles Red Cross also recalled 1,400 suspect blood products that had been improperly released because of the center's "systematic failure" to follow safety testing procedures. The Red Cross in Columbus, Ohio, recalled 376 HIV-reactive blood products that had been shipped to New York, Georgia, Florida, and Switzerland. There was no computer system in place to ensure that headquarters even knew its regions' disposition of possibly contaminated blood.

In March 1988, twenty-four units of blood or blood products were voluntarily recalled for "possible contamination" in Nashville and Washington, D.C. FDA inspectors found that "standard operating procedures were not followed in handling these blood products." Of those recalled units, ten units of plasma intended for fractionation had tested initially reactive for HIV antibodies; some of those units were used in manufacturing. Five units of recovered or salvaged plasma tested positive for hepatitis B surface antigen; four of those units had entered the manufacturing process. Nine units were obtained from donors "who may have been unsuitable according to accepted guidelines," including risk factors for AIDS. Two other units which were not part of the recall had "questionable" HIV antibody test results but were shipped and used for transfusion; follow-up testing of the donors showed them to be HIV negative.

In May 1988, the Red Cross had suspended its plasma business because of FDA's concern about product safety. That six month halt of plasma distribution would be cited in Red Cross's annual report as having "contributed greatly to the $17.7 million deficit incurred to support Blood Services operations, working capital requirements, and fixed asset acquisitions" in fiscal year 1988.

Two months later in July the Red Cross temporarily closed its St. Louis testing laboratories when it learned that the center had issued 264 units with incomplete test results to hospitals or for further manufacture. However, FDA and Red Cross investigations showed "no confirmed HIV antibody positive blood was transfused."

Under threat of federal action, the Red Cross signed an agreement with FDA to clean up its blood regions. The 1988 voluntary agreement called for the Red Cross to "explore the feasibility of alternative systems to the current practice of accepting blood donations from donors temporarily deferred due to repeatedly reactive screening tests" for HIV and hepatitis and to standardize its procedures, update its audits, and install computer systems. The Red Cross was instructed to report back to FDA in sixty days to show evidence that clear lines of authority between its regions and headquarters had been established.

During the summer of 1988, as the Red Cross was chided by the FDA, hearings were held before the Presidential Commission on AIDS. Blood expert and FDA Blood Products Advisory Committee member Professor Ross Eckert spoke of the continued risks to the blood supply. Among them was HTLV-1, a devastating form of leukemia and nerve disease resembling multiple sclerosis. HTLV-1 had been found in ten of nearly 40,000 blood samples drawn from the Red Cross blood centers in eight cities. But like AIDS, HTLV-1 had a long latency period, and the number of victims could not yet be assessed.

Meanwhile, IV drug users continued to give blood. Researchers at Johns Hopkins studying the blood donation activity of nearly 3,000 IV drug users in the Baltimore, Maryland area found that one in four IV drug users had given plasma or blood between 1978 and 1988; one in ten donated between 1987 and 1989.

"Blood is not safe," Eckert said. "Blood banks testing for HIV and hepatitis have high error rates, but such errors are small problems compared with the ongoing casualties resulting from inadequate screening of donors throughout the blood industry."

Recipients of bad blood had little recourse. The industry was effectively shielded from product liability laws. "Why do we exempt blood banks from the tragedies that their services cause when we do not exempt manufacturers of badly designed drugs, aircraft, or lawnmowers?" Eckert asked the commission.

Ross Eckert was accused by blood bankers of creating "unnecessary panic about AIDS." In 1995, Eckert himself would succumb to AIDS. He was a hemophiliac.

Edgar Engleman, director of the Stanford University Blood Bank, told the President's AIDS panel, "The blood bankers blew it. In another ten years, another threat will arise and the same thing will happen all over again. I don't mean to place blame, but to try to find out why."

On December 8, 1989, Washington, D.C. Superior Court judge Richard Salzman issued a breakthrough decision in the matter of *Wilson v. the American Red Cross*. Unlike his judicial peers, who dismissed claims of negligence against the Red Cross, Salzman found that Rita Wilson's claim on behalf of her deceased daughter deserved to be heard by a jury. For the first time, the Red Cross's "standard of care" defense did not protect it from a jury trial. Rather, Salzman found, "Standard of care is a question of fact, a variant of what the reasonably prudent person would do, albeit what a reasonable medical professional would do . . . measured by what they knew at the time. I think professionals understood the potential seriousness of the AIDS epidemic that was about to descend on us, and that some people did not act upon that seriousness as quickly as they could."

Following that decision, the Red Cross opted not to go to trial. It settled the claims brought on behalf of Andrea Wilson for an undisclosed amount and obtained protective orders sealing the sensitive internal Red Cross documents.

The Red Cross's lawyers made another request: they asked Judge Salzman to vacate his decision. They argued that since it had decided to settle, the judge's ruling to allow the case to proceed to trial was moot. As a matter of law, however, Salzman's ruling was important. The Wilson case could be cited by other plaintiff attorneys challenging the Red Cross on its standard of care argument. Judge Salzman agreed to vacate his ruling.

Despite several rulings supporting the Red Cross's standard of care defense, the courts were sufficiently at odds for Ashcraft & Gerel's attorneys to contemplate a court victory in future transfusion-AIDS cases.

For one, the Red Cross's argument against donor disclosure, successfully won in South Carolina and Tennessee, had been more recently patently shot down by two other federal courts. One judge found, "There is not one shred of tangible evidence . . . to substantiate otherwise speculative claims that the blood supply will be jeopardized" by allowing donors to be deposed.

Two important studies published in prestigious medical journals underscored the negligence of the blood industry in the early 1980s. Those studies confirmed what plaintiff lawyers had argued on behalf of their client; namely that direct questioning of donors' sexual lifestyle would not have alienated donors, and that high-risk individuals were continuing to give blood.

In October 1989, Dr. Susan Leitman of the National Institutes of Health and Dr. Fred Darr of the Red Cross in Washington, D.C. published the findings of their collaborative study of HIV-infected donors. The study examined blood tests of individuals who had donated at the D.C. center between July 1985 and December 1988. During that period, the AIDS-specific test was in use, and the risk groups for AIDS were widely known. Leitman and Darr wanted to know whether donors at high risk were actually self-deferring. During the study period, 284 donors tested reactive for AIDS in the Red Cross blood center in D.C. The majority of these HIV-reactive donors had *not* self-deferred. Although 106 were homosexual or bisexual men, they did not believe their behavior put them at high risk for AIDS. All scored abnormally high when their blood was also examined for T-cell count and hepatitis core antibody.

The second significant study that year confirmed Leitman's findings. It also examined direct donor questioning. Dr. A. J. Silvergleid of the Blood Bank of San Bernadino and Riverside (California) Counties joined with colleagues at UCLA's School of Medicine to evaluate the attitude of prospective donors to direct questioning. Silvergleid found that among San Bernadino's donors who were surveyed, ninety percent overwhelmingly supported explicit questioning of high-risk behavior, including sexual practices. Only one percent stated they would stop donating if they were asked such pointed questions. Furthermore, the effect on blood donations was not negative, as the Red Cross had predicted in 1983. On the contrary, donations increased four percent to seven percent at some locations.

The authors concluded, "It is clear from our data that direct questioning is well received by donors, who generally perceive it to be in the interest of greater safety. Concerns about offending donors, the major reason cited for the reluctance of many centers to adopt this approach, was not substantiated by our experience."

Had the Leitman or Silvergleid studies been conducted in the early 1980s, the Red Cross would have had no justifiable basis for rejecting direct donor screening or surrogate testing.

There was also a recent breakthrough ruling that put a crimp in the Red Cross's defense of its practices in the early 1980s. In 1989, the Red Cross's peer, the American Association of Blood Banks, was found liable for $405,000 of a $1.35 million jury award in a transfusion-AIDS case. In 1984, William Snyder, a New Jersey man, had undergone heart surgery; three years later he learned he had acquired AIDS from the transfusion. He sued the Bergen County Blood Center, St. Joseph's Hospital and several doctors, as well as the blood supplier, the AABB. The AABB, Snyder contended, had been negligent in its failure to properly test its blood for HIV. The AABB argued that the surrogate test was unnecessary and too expensive.

Snyder won. The other defendants settled but the blood organization appealed on the basis of qualified immunity contending it was "quasi government [in] nature in regulating blood banks." The Red Cross employed a similar defense as well. In June 1996, the New Jersey Supreme Court would reject AABB's arguments. "Nothing other than AABB's own self-interest and tragically bad judgment prevented [it] from recommending surrogate testing." The ruling held significant implications for the Red Cross, as well: "The foreseeability, not the conclusiveness, of harm suffices to give rise to a duty of care. By 1983, ample evidence supported the conclusion that blood transmitted the AIDS virus. In early 1984, the AABB knew that AIDS was a rapidly spreading, fatal disease and that apparently healthy donors could infect others. The AABB also knew that blood and blood products probably could transmit AIDS and that each infected blood donor could infect many donees. Thus, the AABB knew, or should have known, in 1984 that the risk of AIDS infection from blood transfusions was devastating."

In late 1989 Feldman, Tisi and Peter Vangsnes, another attorney at their firm, accepted Roland Ray's case. They explained to him the kinds of road blocks the Red Cross would put up and that the Red Cross was as formidable an adversary as it was an unlikely defendant in the public's mind. Roland assured his attorneys that he and Janet had no illusions. He and his wife had come by way of shock, rage and grief to see justice served. They wanted to bring their case before ordinary people like themselves. There was more at stake than his own life, Roland said. People had to know the truth.

If it could happen to him, it could happen to anyone.

CHAPTER EIGHT

TICKING TIME BOMBS

1990

No patient has ever been known to have acquired hepatitis B or AIDS as a result of a procedural or technical or computer error on the part of Red Cross.

Red Cross statement
July 1990

Of all Heather Michaels's dolls, her favorite was Jillie Ann. She named Jillie Ann after her father, Jim, because, "Jillie has blue eyes like my daddy." Heather liked to sit on her grandmother Jewelle's lap and, with Jillie Ann, "drive" the old Chevy up and down the driveway. Even when she lost sight in her left eye from AIDS-related complications, Heather insisted she and Jillie Ann continue driving, but Jewelle did most of the steering.

When Heather felt too sick to sit in the car, she'd say, "Let's quit it for a while, Granny." When the shooting pains in her legs became unbearable and her body started shaking, she sat on her bed and rocked Jillie Ann. Sometimes she would draw in her coloring book. Or she would ask her father to play a KISS or Mariah Carey album. Holly and Hailey would dance around the bed in pink tutus while Heather moved her upper body to the music.

At various intervals the girls suffered outbreaks of skin rashes, and they did not go to school; tutors came to the house. When the skin condition completely subsided, they returned to their classes. Holly, in particular, adored school, and her teachers adored her. No one knew about their illness, not even the girls.

One night an evening news show broadcast a special on AIDS. At that time, Holly was suffering an allergic skin reaction, and her body was covered with a mosaic of reddish brown blotches. A man whose face was similarly marked was being interviewed. Holly's gaze was fixed on the AIDS patient. The camera then scanned the assortment of pills he was taking.

"Daddy," Holly said, "those pills look like what we take."

Jim had never lied to his daughters, and he wasn't about to now. They had begun asking questions about why they were sick so much of the time. The trips to Charlottesville to see Dr. Saulsbury had become more frequent. By now, each had a "portocath" implanted under her skin. The catheter entered a main artery so that Jim could administer their medication without repeatedly puncturing their skin with a needle.

Hailey, Heather, and Holly were about seven years old when Jim, Debby, and Jewelle sat them down on the couch in the living room and Jim told them they were "HIV positive." He explained that they had been infected with a disease, a virus. It wasn't their fault, he said. It was just something that happened.

The girls listened solemnly. Then Holly asked, "How did it happen, Daddy?"

Jim said they'd caught this virus from a blood transfusion when they were little babies. They needed that blood so they would live. But it was, Jim explained, "bad blood, and now you got a bad virus."

Jewelle watched her granddaughters' faces as Jim told them they would probably not live to grow up. She and Jim had always spoken to them about Jesus. Now Jim was telling them they would go to live with Jesus in heaven.

Hailey asked if he could come, too.

Jim said someday they would all be together.

The girls remained quiet for a few moments. Then Heather turned to Jewelle. "Granny," she said, "when I go to heaven I want you to take care of Jillie Ann. Because I will be back, Granny. I *will.*"

Stephen Sims, deputy staff director for the House Subcommittee on Oversight and Investigations of the House Commerce and Energy Committee, and a former foreign affairs analyst for the CIA, thought that he had lost the ability to be surprised. He had spent sixteen years with Oversight, twelve of which under its chairman, Congressman John Dingell, navigating inquiries through the mire of federal agencies that had at one point or other been under investigation; these included the Securities and Exchange Commission, the Federal Communications Commission, and FDA. Sims had become all too familiar with the friendly back-slapping that developed between watchdog agencies and the industries they were supposed to monitor.

The revolving door between government and special interests maintained the status quo.

By 1990, Sims had an impressive track record steering explosive issues through political mazes: phony birth control pills trafficked out of South America; drug rings that involved big money payoffs and prostitution and implicated federal employees; scientific fraud at prestigious universities; contraband goods; and FBI stings—plots and subplots that were far stranger than fiction.

The FDA was a particularly tight clique. The products it regulated made up, after all, about one-quarter of the Gross National Product. There was a lot of power there. But in the process he believed the public got short shrift.

Sims knew only peripherally about the blood supply. Even the most informed members of Congress seemed to have scant knowledge of just what blood bankers did. Nobody seemed to pay them much attention. He had only recently begun following the blood scandal among the nation's 20,000 hemophiliacs. Half had already shown symptoms of AIDS. It was tragic, but the hemophiliac community was a relatively small one. It did not have the kind of national scope Sims needed to put before a Dingell subcommittee.

What caught his attention was a series on the Red Cross in the *Philadelphia Inquirer* that began in the summer of 1989. Like most Americans, Steve Sims thought of the Red Cross as a virtually sacred institution. If you couldn't rely on the Red Cross, what could you rely on? He had no idea that the charity was the leader in the multibillion-dollar blood industry.

The Red Cross's plasma business had grown so disproportionately that its revenues were no longer substantially related to its tax-exempt standing. Commercial plasma brokers were protesting the Red Cross's tax privileges. H. Edward Matveld of Alpha Therapeutics testified during a June 1987 Congressional inquiry, "The American Red Cross is perceived by the public as a benevolent group of volunteers who make the donation of blood as painless and socially significant as possible. The public is not generally aware of its incredible wealth."

Sims was intrigued. He obtained documentation cited in the newspaper series, and he read *And the Band Played On* by Randy Shilts, which chronicled the early spread of the AIDS epidemic through-out the world. What struck Sims were FDA inspection reports of Red Cross blood centers from 1988 and 1989. The Red Cross was in overt violation not only of the 1988 federal Voluntary Agreement, but of its own institutional procedures.

Its blood regions were, Sims thought, "ticking time bombs."

Since October 1989, FDA records had shown that blood collection agencies had recalled more than 370,000 units of blood and plasma that should not have been released. In 1989 alone, the Red Cross had been forced to recall 5,700 units of blood and blood components that had been improperly tested for AIDS and hepatitis. That did not necessarily mean all unsuitable units had been caught in time. Some of those recalls involved products distributed long ago. Given the timely need for blood, chances were that questionable units had long been transfused, or manufactured into hemophiliac clotting products.

That same year alone the FDA had logged 1,000 blood bank errors but had taken little or no punitive action. In the prior four years, despite an horrendous blood industry track record, the FDA had imposed sanctions only 33 times. In early 1990, blood banks had already reported 29,586 "mishaps."

Sims also learned that in January 1988, the FDA had finally required that AIDS tests be done on all donated blood. Previously AIDS testing had merely been a "recommendation," which did not carry the weight of law. However, scores of units of untested blood remained in back inventories; no law required blood banks to test their stock.

While FDA had been successful in uncovering abuses, it had not convinced Red Cross to take corrective action. Here was a revered organization, well endowed in resources, that was operating in such chaos that it had been subject to federal intervention.

For the first time in nearly two decades, Steve Sims was surprised.

Implicating the nation's most respected charity in what looked at best like negligence, at worst criminal activity, was not a task for the fainthearted. The Red Cross held tremendous sway. Its Board of Directors was a veritable social, political, and economic Who's Who, as it had been throughout its entire history. For this investigation, he knew, he would have to have his "ducks in a row."

Certain problems were apparent from the start. The Red Cross was a very insular, decentralized entity that had been handled with kid gloves by the FDA. As a result, there was still no standardization of practices, no clear line of authority from headquarters to the regions. Sims would later recall, "The power over blood collection in the regions was held by the same person who supervised the swim lessons. You had a sophisticated biomedical operation that was being run by do-gooders who were interested in giving out coffee and donuts to disaster relief workers."

By the time Sims walked into Dingell's office, early 1990, he had a thick folder of incriminating evidence. He placed the stack of papers on Dingell's desk and said, "Boss, I think we should investigate the Red Cross."

The congressman put down his pen and leaned back in his chair. Sims could see he was taken aback, but interested. So Sims briefed him: bad blood, blood feuds, blood money. There seemed to be no accountability. The FDA was "a paper tiger." It had no authority to fine blood banks that violated federal safety standards, and its suspension-for-cause record was abominable. The FDA's hands-off and the Red Cross's arrogance were exposing the public to lethal health risks.

But when push came to shove, the Red Cross was a lot more powerful than FDA. "If the FDA declared war, the Red Cross would easily win," Sims told Dingell.

He saw Dingell was hooked.

"Keep me informed," Dingell told him, then returned to his own stack of papers.

Sims would later recall the implicit warning couched in that approval: "Be careful, and for heaven's sake, don't do something crazy."

Steve Sims expected that the Red Cross would not be pleased with the subcommittee's interest. The organization had its own corporate culture, a mindset that was particularly resistant to change. It seemed to have a sense of entitlement as the "unimpeachable good guys."

What surprised him most was the Red Cross's outrage at being questioned.

It was Sims's practice to meet face-to-face with the heads of agencies, companies, or organizations that would be facing public scrutiny. At a closed meeting at the Red Cross headquarters, he informed senior administrators and representatives from the regions that they had very serious problems that had to be fixed. There was going to be a subcommittee investigation. That meant public hearings.

Sims explained to the Red Cross officers what their lives were going to be like for the next several months, maybe a year, maybe longer.

The Red Cross had only recently gone through a reorganization, following the resignation of longtime president Richard Schubert. The former vice chairman of Bethlehem Steel, Dick Schubert had become president of the Red Cross in January 1983, just as the AIDS issue was coming to the fore. At his departure, the Red Cross credited him with launching a "major AIDS public education program."

Red Cross chairman George Moody, president of the Security Pacific Corporation in Los Angeles, had created a special team to manage the organization until a new president was chosen. Alfred Katz, now senior medical director, and Arnie deBeaufort, from finance and administration, were among those selected to report to Blood Services vice president Leweylls Barker. Dr. William Miller was named group vice president of biomedical operations.

Sims welcomed the Red Cross's cooperation, but he made it clear he was going to forge ahead, with or without its help. "We can either do this working together, or if you want to fight us, we will do it against your opposition."

There was no evidence that the Red Cross attempted to use its politically powerful connections to thwart the subcommittee's investigation. It was, Sims observed, "a perception."

On May 12, 1990, Ryan White, the hemophiliac teenager who, for millions of Americans, had put a human face on AIDS, died. Barbara Bush and Michael Jackson were among over 1,000 mourners at his funeral in Indianapolis. Phil Donahue, on whose show Ryan had appeared, was a pallbearer. Elton John sang. So did a twelve-girl swing choir, which chose "That's What Friends Are For," the song that had come to symbolize the AIDS fight.

Ryan was eighteen.

With blood-borne AIDS thrust into the media spotlight, the Dingell subcommittee hearings could not have opened at a more propitious time.

"The bad news," Congressman John Dingell told a packed room, "is that the American Red Cross, which collects over half of all the whole blood in the United States, has had serious and persistent problems with its procedures for testing and keeping track of this blood. According to inspection reports by the Food and Drug Administration and the Red Cross's own internal reports, various Red Cross collection centers have released infected blood, mixed up records, violated AIDS testing procedures, and failed to deter infected or undesirable donors." Moreover, the FDA's inspection of Red Cross National Headquarters found that "Red Cross blood collection centers were not even complying with the Red Cross's own standard operating procedures, this in apparent violation of the September 1988 agreement between the Red Cross and the FDA."

Dingell expressed bewilderment at a significant discrepancy between a recent Red Cross public statement and information from CDC. On July 10, the Red Cross had issued a press release indicating that "only six cases of transfusion AIDS have been reported since the testing and screening [of blood] have been instituted."

"Notwithstanding the problems that the Red Cross has experienced in keeping track of donors and units of blood after they have been tested, the Red Cross statement was somewhat startling to the committee," Dingell said. "The CDC monthly HIV/AIDS report shows that so far this year, 76 people have been added to the list of transfusion-AIDS cases each month. Why the discrepancy?"

The blood industry's failure in the 1980s to address transfusion AIDS prompted impassioned dialogue as the hearing opened. Dr. Marcus Conant, the University of California AIDS specialist and co-chair of the California AIDS Leadership Committee, condemned both government and industry for failing to deal head-on with the blood problem. Conant pointed out that "between twelve and twenty-two thousand Americans were infected with the HIV virus as a direct result of blood transfusion because of a failure of blood banks to screen out high-risk donors, the failure of the blood industry to accurately disseminate information, the failure of the division of Biologicals of the FDA to demand minimum standards of donor evaluation and product screening, and a failure of the CDC to demand accountability of the blood industry and the blood regulators." By the time the AIDS test became widely available in March 1985, some 15,000 Americans had already been infected with blood-borne HIV. Most of these tragedies could have been avoided, Conant said, with proper donor screening and surrogate testing.

Georgia Congressman Roy Rowland asked Conant about a particularly early decision made by blood bankers. Rowland, also a physician, cited a memo by Joseph Bove, chair of the industry's

Transfusion Transmitted Diseases Committee, on which the Red Cross served. Rowland read aloud parts of Bove's January 24, 1983 letter to the committee that referenced the 1982 transfusion case of an infant in Texas. That case, Bove wrote, "increases the probability that AIDS may be spread by blood." But he continued with a warning: "We do not want anything that we do now to be interpreted by society or by legal authorities as agreeing with the concept, as yet unproven, that AIDS can be spread by blood."

Rowland told the Dingell committee, "There is pretty plain language here. It seems to be that AIDS is probably spread by transfusion. In most cases it is virtually certain. But the blood bankers did not want to really acknowledge that."

He asked for Conant's interpretation.

Conant replied: "Bove doesn't want anything that they do to be construed by society or lawyers as agreeing with the concept [of transfusion AIDS]. And then he says, 'I hope that we are equipped psychologically to continue to act together.' He has been in contact with Dr. [Fred] Katz [of the Red Cross] and Dr. Menitove and believes that the 'three of us can act together to work out whatever new problems may arise.' That sounds like collusion."

Subsequent testimony by Professor Ross Eckert of the FDA's Blood Advisory Board and Stanford University's Edgar Engleman described how the priorities of the early 1980s imperiled recipients of blood products. The blood industry was, they claimed, more concerned with image and economics than public health.

FDA senior investigator Mary Carden who had been tracking Red Cross read off a litany of violations recorded during inspections from January to early July 1990. At Red Cross centers nationwide, standard operating procedure for handling error and accident reports had not been reviewed, in some cases, since July 1981 and were severely inadequate. No time frame had been established for submitting reports to the FDA. There was no provision for analyses of error reports, no means of assuring that donors testing positive for infectious diseases were deferred. There was still no computer system in place to adequately track donors and recipients, this in violation of federal Look-Back requirements. The FDA had taken an unprecedented step and revoked the Albany center's license, after finding 63 violations resulting in the release of HIV-reactive blood.

The FDA was distressed by ongoing problems in Farmington, Connecticut. There, deferred donors who had tested HIV reactive in 1985 were not placed in the deferral file until 1988. One donor who had tested reactive in November 1986 was not deferred until February 1987. In the interim, products from that donated blood were released and distributed.

In Dedham, Massachusetts, about 500 donors who repeatedly tested reactive for hepatitis were placed into a "surveillance" category, rather than deferred. Blood from seven of those donors was released. In 1986, twenty-five products had been manufactured from HIV-reactive blood and distributed.

But among centers in chronic violation, the most remiss was Washington D.C. The FDA found that in over 230 cases of transfusion AIDS dating as far back as 1983, only four had been reported to the Red Cross headquarters as of July 1990.

D.C. was also dragging its heels on tracing 300 HIV-reactive donors who had given blood prior to 1985. By mid-1990, few had been notified. One donor, who had been implicated in five transfusion-AIDS cases, had given blood 79 times.

In the Heart of Illinois region, 350 units of plasma that raised questions in liver enzyme and HIV assays had been released in 1988. Headquarters had known of the error, but did not recall the products until May 1990, or later. Bacterial contamination in Penn-Jersey resulted in adverse reactions. In the Appalachia region, salmonella contamination of blood products led to a recall of recovered plasma.

Congress learned that the Red Cross had not even reported to the FDA, 386 errors and accidents involving the release of HIV-reactive or otherwise tainted blood. Those mishaps had not even been reviewed by the Red Cross's own regulatory affairs.

Investigator Mary Carden, who had been with the FDA since 1978, had found most regional blood bankers "prompt in providing indications that they've already corrected the deficiency or are going to do the best they can. In the case of [the] inspection of the American Red Cross at National Headquarters," she told the subcommittee, "that type of attitude did not prevail. There were no promises of corrective action during the inspection. I did not see any expression of concern at all from anyone that I dealt with."

When Carden asked Red Cross personnel about their failure to report errors to FDA in a timely manner, one employee indicated this was "not [her] first priority." Another stated that the "situation has been worse." At one meeting, Carden was asked to leave the room while senior officials discussed "if they would like to respond at that time."

The Red Cross's attitude was, Carden said, "highly unusual."

D.C.'s former director, Dr. Fred Darr, told the FDA inspectors that he had repeatedly complained about work overload. "[He] could not do what needed to be done" regarding Look-Back cases. The FDA noted a memo from Darr to the Red Cross associate general counsel Karen Shoos Lipton in which he expressed concern that a donor to the Columbus [Ohio] Red Cross was positive. That donor had previously given blood in Washington, D.C. and had been implicated in a number of AIDS cases. Yet he was not in the National Referred Donor Registry.

When Carden asked Darr how an HIV-reactive unit which had been quarantined and tagged in a bag for disposal had ended up back on the lab shelf, Darr said he thought it was "sabotage." In his view, problems within the regions "took precedence over the Look-Back and TAA [transfusion-associated AIDS] case investigations." Other staff complained to the FDA that "the only TAA cases getting any attention were the ones involved in litigation."

One of the most egregious violators was the Portland, Oregon blood center, where HIV-reactive blood was mislabeled and shipped out for transfusion, blood products were made from permanently deferred donors, and quarantine procedures were not being followed. Oregon congressman Ron Wyden, whose constituents were hit hardest by those violations, was later interviewed by *60 Minutes.* He stated, "I think it's just tragic that the Red Cross, which is regarded by millions as essentially the organization that helps maintain life or death in this country, has been very deficient in some of its safety practices."

At the hearings, the Red Cross assured the FDA it was taking steps to correct its deficiencies. A Red Cross spokesperson defending the Washington, D.C. center told the *Washington Post,* "In the course of our own inspections, there was *no evidence* found that any blood that tested positive after 1985 was improperly released" [emphasis added].

That summer, the Red Cross began a major reorganization aimed at reining in its local blood centers. Following the Dingell hearings, Dr. Jeffrey McCullough, a well-respected physician from the University of Minnesota, was named senior vice president of Biomedical Services. He would be responsible for managing the restructuring. Blood Services would operate separately from disaster relief. Each region would be headed by a principal officer (PO). Unlike previous regional managers, the PO would report directly to McCullough. The plan was for the POs to be physicians.

At a media briefing in the summer of 1990, McCullough explained, "It is essential for all blood centers to recognize the public trust and make decisions in a more public forum, rather than purely a medical/technical format. It's not appropriate for a dozen doctors to sit around and determine blood policy."

As for the safety of the blood supply, McCullough insisted, "I believe that the Red Cross is operating a very effective and very safe blood program."

On July 16, three days after the Dingell hearings, Ashcraft & Gerel attorneys Mike Feldman, Chris Tisi, and Peter Vangsnes filed a class action suit in D.C. Superior Court on behalf of the 235 transfusion-AIDS victims of the Red Cross's D.C. center. The class action representatives were Roland and Janet Ray. The suit charged the Red Cross with negligence in failing to use surrogate tests, and failing to screen out high-risk donors.

The suit did more than cite Red Cross negligence. *Ray v. the American Red Cross* alleged, "The Red Cross colluded and conspired with the AABB [American Association of Blood Banks] and the CCBC [Council of Community Blood Centers] to actively prevent the widespread adoption of surrogate testing for HIV. The Red Cross intentionally and willfully blocked the use of surrogate tests for HIV on a nationwide basis despite specific knowledge that AIDS was transmissible by blood, that high-risk donors continued to donate despite requests to self-defer, and that the use of surrogate tests would screen a high percentage of HIV-infected persons from the blood supply so as to save the lives of the recipients."

Only days before his attorney filed the lawsuit, Roland had called his children, Wayne, eleven, and Sandra, sixteen, into the living room. He told them that during his surgery six years ago, he had had a blood transfusion. He thought the transfusion would save his life; instead, he had been infected with bad blood. He now had AIDS.

Wayne and Sandra clung to him, crying. He assured them that Janet and the baby, Emily, were okay. "As long as God needs me to be alive to take care of you," he said, "I will be here."

Despite its brave face before the public, the Red Cross knew it was in trouble. Transfusion-AIDS cases like Roland Ray's were coming down the pike. The FDA was still finding widespread Red Cross violations at blood centers. Congress was breathing down its neck. If ever the Red Cross needed its own "Angel of Mercy," it was now.

The Red Cross perceived its salvation in the person of Elizabeth Hanford Dole. It was a marriage made in public relations heaven.

CHAPTER NINE

A SEAT AT THE TABLE

The positive use of power is a good thing. You've got to be able to have that seat at the table.

Elizabeth Dole

To hear Elizabeth Dole tell it, her meteoric rise to the echelons of Washington, D.C.'s power elite was sheer serendipity, a metamorphosis from southern belle to Cabinet secretary. Her success appeared to be a perplexing mystery.

In reality, Elizabeth Hanford Dole, who served six presidents and was the only woman in U.S. history to hold two separate Cabinet posts in two administrations, had been preparing herself for prominence since she was a child.

"She was never satisfied," her mother, Mary Cathey Hanford, told *Life* magazine. "She always wanted to be at the top."

Mary Elizabeth Hanford was born on July 29, 1936, of southern gentry, the youngest child of a wealthy florist and a devout Christian mother. She grew up in the quaint, prosperous town of Salisbury, North Carolina in a stately three-story Tudor home. Mrs. Dole, who nicknamed herself "Liddy," had an idyllic childhood. There were all the pleasures of a privileged upbringing: horseback riding, ballet and tap-dancing lessons, tennis, piano, summers in the mountains or at the shore, a beloved pet Chihuahua, adventurous family vacations by rail to the West Coast and Canada, cotillions, and a debutante ball.

In her autobiography, *Unlimited Partners,* written with her husband, Robert Dole, she described herself as "a serious child and eager to please." Her ambition and compulsiveness surfaced early. As a flower girl at weddings, she would scatter flower petals at exactly the same intervals. She held her first elected office in the third grade, when she started a bird club and was elected its president. Three years later, she deliberately tested different handwriting styles before deciding on the one she would use.

"She was overly conscientious and wanted to please so bad," her second-grade teacher recalled in the biography *Elizabeth Dole, Public Servant.*

Early on, Mrs. Dole also paid meticulous attention to image. Her high school classmates viewed her as a glamorous, impeccably dressed young woman whose eyeglasses were tastefully chosen to match her outfits. At Duke University, she adhered verbatim to the coed handbook, à la Emily Post: "A Duchess should have the tact and good judgment to know when the occasion requires her to be serious and when to be gay, when to dress up and when to be casual. Everything she does is in good taste and up to the highest standards."

She was class president and May Queen, graduated Phi Beta Kappa, and was designated Duke's 1958 "Leader of the Year."

"Old curiosity about remote places and lifestyles," as Liddy Dole put it, drew her to Harvard University. While earning a master's degree in teaching and government, Mrs. Dole worked at the law library. In 1960, she landed in Washington and got a job in the office of North Carolina Senator B. Everett Jordan. Bill Cochrane, a former aide to the senator, told the *Washington Monthly*, "She walked through the door, she didn't have an appointment, and we hired her that afternoon. Phi Beta Kappa at Duke and Queen of the May, she was extremely qualified."

And she was driven. From the start, Mrs. Dole sought out mentors among prominent women in government. She dated "men with promising political futures," Suzanne Rodgers Busch, a staff member in Senator Jordan's office and former housemate of Mrs. Dole's, recalled. Friends used to say that Liddy Hanford was either going to marry into the White House or get elected herself.

Nineteen-sixty was a presidential campaign year. Mrs. Dole managed to get aboard vice-presidential candidate Lyndon B. Johnson's whistlestop train tour of the South. But her Republican father did not take kindly to his daughter's pitch for the Democrats. She mollified him, explaining, "Now, Dad, it will be perfectly all right. It's just a learning experience. It doesn't mean anything." That philosophy would enable her to shift seamlessly from Democratic to Republican administrations, as seamlessly adapting her politics to conform to the mindset in residence.

In 1962, Mrs. Dole enrolled in Harvard Law School, one of only two dozen women in a class of 550. Her parents were alarmed. At age 26, their only daughter could be a spinster. Didn't she want to be a wife, mother, and hostess for a husband? Mrs. Dole wanted all that and more. "After all," she explained, "it was my life, my little red wagon."

At Harvard, she was elected president of the International Law Club and class secretary, a lifetime position.

Washington drew her, she said, "like a magnet." After a brief stint at the Department of Health, Education and Welfare and a year as a public defender, Mrs. Dole landed a job in the White House Office of Consumer Affairs. The new job placed her in the middle of a burgeoning consumer movement. Her boss, well-known consumer advocate Betty Furness, told the *Washington Monthly* that Mrs. Dole seemed to be "right with us" on pro-consumer issues. When Richard Nixon brought to the White House a decidedly more big-business orientation, most of Mrs. Dole's colleagues fled. She, however, muted her pro-consumer approach and remained. Subsequently she developed a close relationship with the new office director, Virginia Knauer, whom she came to view as a mentor and surrogate mother.

"Whether Elizabeth changed her mind or changed her colors, I don't know," despaired the now-deceased Furness. One thing Mrs. Dole did change was her registration—from Democrat to Independent.

In 1973, Knauer recommended Mrs. Dole for an appointment to the Federal Trade Commission (FTC), the agency responsible for consumer protection and monitoring business practices. Nixon agreed, but Congress viewed Mrs. Dole more as White House insider than consumer advocate. Not one to take no for an answer, she quickly orchestrated what she called a "constructive dialogue" with consumer advocates. Her efforts resulted in an avalanche of endorsements from consumer leaders, two dozen state attorneys general, a number of journalists, and North Carolina senators Sam Ervin and Jesse Helms. Testifying before the Senate confirmation committee, she railed against consumer abuses and "giant conglomerate firms," promising a "renewed consumer-oriented thrust" at the FTC. Her new position was, she explained, a "logical extension of my earlier work on behalf of individuals victimized by discrimination or economic abuse."

On December 3, 1973, Mrs. Dole was sworn in as Federal Trade Commissioner from a hospital bed at Georgetown University, where she was recovering from an injury after a car accident.

During her tenure on the FTC, Mrs. Dole was widely perceived as a strong consumer advocate. She stood up to big business on issues like false advertising and full disclosure to consumers. She was also vigorous on antitrust. Espousing the principle that the best market for consumers is one in which "there are many sellers, none of which has any significant market share," she opposed most mergers that came before the FTC.

She did, however, make a successful personal merger. In the spring of 1972, her mentor from Nixon's consumer bureau directed Elizabeth Hanford to the office of Senator Robert Dole. Her purpose was to lobby on a consumer issue. Impressed with her charm and good looks, the newly divorced Republican senator from Kansas jotted this lobbyist's name on his blotter. It took the senator, who was head of the Republican Party and one of the most powerful men on Capitol Hill, several months to work up the courage to call. Meanwhile, she kept her eyes open for other prospects, among them an eligible congressman from Mississippi. But by the summer of 1974, with Bob Dole in a reelection campaign for the Senate, their lives began to merge. There were daily telephone calls from the Kansas campaign trail. Soon after winning reelection, Senator Dole proposed. They were married on December 6, 1975. The union of the two political powerhouses prompted FTC counsel Ronald A. Bloch to suggest that the marriage might constitute a violation of federal antitrust laws. She was 36, he was 49. The charming and successful Elizabeth Dole and her handsome war-hero husband quickly earned the distinction of Washington's "power couple."

Just eight months later, Elizabeth Dole's husband was chosen as Gerald Ford's vice presidential running mate.

In Bob Dole, Liddy had met her perfect match: "We had so much in common, not least of all careers that were distinct but in some ways overlapping." The senator recalled, "We speak the same language. We share the same passion for public service."

Jeanne Eberhart Dubovfsky, a law school colleague of Mrs. Dole's and a former Colorado Supreme Court Justice, spoke to a *New Yorker* reporter about Liddy Hanford's marriage to Senator Dole. "[She was] very conscious of the limits that were placed on women then.

She thought that to be successful you'd have to be the wife of the President. . . . When I heard she had married Dole, I thought it was very funny." Tanya Melich, a former Republican Party official and author of *The Republican War against Women,* observed that by marrying Bob Dole, the politically moderate Elizabeth became more acceptable to the Republican right, which was gaining prominence in Washington.

After her marriage, Mrs. Dole changed her registration from Independent to Republican and avidly hit the campaign trail on behalf of her husband.

Her assiduous campaigning did not charm everyone. California congressman John Moss, head of the House Commerce Oversight Committee, called for an investigation into whether Mrs. Dole had violated the nonpartisan nature of her post by campaigning for the Republican ticket. Although the Library of Congress found that Mrs. Dole had not violated federal ethics and conflict of interest rules, Congressman Moss declared, "The partisan political activities of Mrs. Dole are absolutely inconsistent with the quasi-judicial nature of her responsibilities as a commissioner." In late September, 1976, Mrs. Dole took a discreet leave of absence from the FTC. Three years later, she resigned from the FTC to support the senator's first bid for the presidency. "How could I sit out one of the great experiences of my husband's life, virtually saying to him, 'Good luck, Bob, and I'll see you when it's over'?" she responded, when criticized by women's advocates.

"From the first day she went out on the trail, she had that natural ability," said Charles Black, Republican political consultant, in a *Washington Monthly* interview. "She probably did more good for Bob Dole than he did for himself." Her husband joked that he withdrew from the race when Elizabeth passed him in the polls. He decided to seek reelection to the Senate.

The Republican victory in the fall of 1980 ushered in a new era of glamour and social ambiance on the Washington scene. Gone were the folksy, populist ways of President Jimmy Carter. High fashion, limousines, fine dining, and elegant parties reigned. Elizabeth Dole, who was named to the Reagan transition team, was a darling of the D.C. glamour set. Speculation was high that she would be appointed to a Cabinet post. Instead, Reagan named her Assistant to the President for Public Liaison, the first woman to hold a top-level White House position. She became gatekeeper to the Oval Office, deciding which constituent groups—labor, women, minorities, industry—gained an audience with the President. Mrs. Dole saw her role as rallying the public around the Reagan agenda, and to "neutralize opposition at the grassroots level," as she put it.

Succeeding in the Reagan administration meant being a friend to corporate America. Mrs. Dole abandoned her championship of consumer issues and spent her time courting industry. Her enthusiastic advocacy of business prompted David Stockman, former Reagan budget director, to write in *The Triumph of Politics* that Mrs. Dole "practically tackled and hog-tied" White House Chief of Staff James Baker to prevent Stockman from eliminating a business tax loophole.

As the Reagan administration faced accusations that its budget cuts hurt the poor and women, Elizabeth Dole became Reagan's "front woman." She was named to the White House Coordinating Council for Women and headed up a newly created "Task Force on Legal Equality for Women," Reagan's counterpoint to the Equal Rights Amendment. She ardently spoke of a "quiet revolution," a "tidal wave of women coming into the work force."

The task force was a "sham," according to Justice Department participant Barbara Honegger. Women's advocates such as Ann F. Lewis, political director of the Democratic National Committee, slammed the Reagan women's initiatives, calling them a "public relations reaction to what is clearly a genuine, substantive problem." By and large, though, Mrs. Dole was off the hook. "Maybe we expected more from her than it was possible for her to give," Patricia Reuss, legislative director of the Women's Equity Action League, told the *New York Times*.

At about this time Mrs. Dole experienced what she described as a "spiritual awakening." In her autobiography, she wrote that she was blessed with a "beautiful marriage and a challenging career," but still she faced "spiritual starvation." She prayed and was blessed: "God led me to people and experiences that transformed my life." When President Reagan asked her to join his Cabinet as Transportation Secretary, Mrs. Dole turned not to her political advisers, but to her spiritual counselors. Principal among them was Jennifer Dorn, a member of her Christian fellowship group and an aide to Republican Senator Mark Hatfield (from Oregon). Jenna Dorn advised her to accept the nomination. She told Mrs. Dole, "Think what it would mean for women."

Mrs. Dole was approved by the Senate on a vote of 97–0. On February 7, 1983, she became the first woman to head the Department of Transportation (DOT). The agency over which Mrs. Dole would reign for the next four and a half years claimed 100,000 employees and a budget of $27 billion. She named Jenna Dorn her special assistant.

Early on, Mrs. Dole showed a talent for public relations. She dubbed herself the "Safety Secretary," and her goal was "Safety in all forms of transportation." One morning she staged a photo opportunity for the press by standing in the DOT parking lot with a stop sign, spot checking her employees to see if they were wearing their safety belts. She launched a number of high-visibility initiatives, including a requirement for center-mounted rear taillights, implementation of random drug testing of DOT employees, state mandatory seat belt laws, and air bags in automobiles, which had been ordered by the Supreme Court but for which she took credit. "I could think of no greater satisfaction than knowing my efforts might contribute to the saving of lives," she recalled.

In a town where image was as potent as position, Mrs. Dole courted the press, and they adored her. *Life* magazine called her "sweet as shoofly pie." *Harper's Bazaar* named her one of the country's ten most influential women. *Fortune* called her "a charmer with impeccable manners" who was also an "astute political operator."

Part of that astuteness was Mrs. Dole's acuity in selecting key advisers, whom *Fortune* referred to as her "armada." Tazewell Eller, an aviation lawyer then on Mrs. Dole's staff, later recalled, "It soon became clear that her public image and the public perception of the department were the predominant factors in all decision-making." Aides were chosen as much for their loyalty as their competence. The nucleus was Jenna Dorn and Mari Maseng. Dorn, who Mrs. Dole referred to as "family," would become associate deputy secretary at DOT and head of a newly created Office of Commercial Space Transportation. Michael Goldfarb, who became chief-of-staff for the Federal Aviation Administration (FAA) and would later serve as a key adviser to Mrs. Dole, was also at the Commercial Space Transportation office.

Of all her advisers, Mrs. Dole had the most in common with Mari Maseng. In 1983, Maseng left the White House to accompany Mrs. Dole to DOT, where she was named Assistant Secretary for public affairs. They met on the 1976 campaign trail, when Maseng was a reporter for the *Charleston Evening Post*. A fellow southerner with an impressive talent for making the right connections, Maseng became staff director for Senator Bob Dole's abortive 1980 presidential campaign, and then moved on to the Reagan-Bush campaign, where she was a media strategist. While Mrs. Dole lobbied constituency groups for Reagan's economic agenda, Maseng wrote the President's speeches. In 1985, Beatrice Foods, a worldwide marketer of foods and consumer products, offered Maseng a position as a vice president, but subsequent corporate reorganization sent her back to the White House to head the Office of Public Liaison, Mrs. Dole's old stomping ground.

Mrs. Dole's inner sanctum tightly controlled her image. "Liddy prepared for things so there would be no surprises," said her old classmate Dubovfsky of Mrs. Dole's penchant for control. "That's the difference between her and other people who appear like her. It may seem effortless, but it's not." Don Byrne, former associate editor of the transport industry's *Traffic World* recalled that during her nearly five-year tenure at DOT, she never held a general press conference. The Q-and-A period was restricted to subjects that had been predetermined. Reporters who diverged from the agenda were "frozen out."

A close examination of Mrs. Dole's performance at DOT revealed more style than substance, a Secretary who made grand gestures with little follow-through, who was adept at "quick fixes" but remiss at addressing more complex, often perilous situations.

One of the more embarrassing moments occurred on December 16, 1984, when Mrs. Dole invited dozens of reporters to Edwards Air Force Base to witness a remote-control jet flight. The Boeing jet was powered by a new fuel designed to prevent the fiery explosions attendant with plane crashes. She billed the "Controlled Impact Demonstration" in the Mojave Desert as the culmination of a five-year, $11.8 million effort by the FAA and NASA to improve the "crash worthiness" of aircraft and save passenger lives. But the jet, with its two dummies, exploded in flames on impact. Dole ducked out after the disaster, leaving her deputy to deal with the fallout.

The airline industry under Dole's tenure suffered some of the worst mishaps in its history. There were a series of spectacular air disasters and near misses, including a close call between President Reagan's helicopter and a private plane over the skies in California. The year 1985 turned out to be the worst one for accidents and deaths in aviation history. Five hundred and twenty-eight people were killed in separate accidents. As a result of deregulation, there were more planes in the sky, and double the number of airlines in the business than there were prior to her term. But the numbers of air traffic controllers and FAA inspectors were drastically reduced. But Mrs. Dole refused to hire more controllers and inspectors until Congress forced her hand. Then she publicly took credit for the increases.

With the industry and DOT under fire, Mrs. Dole launched a highly publicized effort to clean up the skies. She announced a $12 billion program to modernize the National Airspace System, which had, in fact, been launched by her predecessor. The program was, she said, the "most complex nonmilitary program of its kind since Project Apollo put a man on the moon." Its goal: to modernize the air traffic system. According to Douglas Feaver, the *Washington Post* journalist who covered DOT issues, the program was widely regarded "as one of government's larger failures that cost the taxpayers a lot of money." Predestined for failure, the program has been plagued by cost overruns, inept management, and contractor problems.

Mrs. Dole's management prompted the chairs of both the House and Senate aviation subcommittees to introduce bills in 1988 to separate the FAA from DOT. The bills, one House staffer recalled, were an "indication of how frustrated members of Congress were about her interference with the FAA. It was viewed as a very serious matter by Congress."

Secretary Dole did pull off a rather spectacular privatization venture, which transferred two major Washington metropolitan area airports, Washington National and Dulles International, from federal to regional control. She recalled the genesis of the idea as late night "pillow talk" with her husband, who said it was a pipe dream. Mrs. Dole took on the challenge. The airport deal, recalled a key Senate staffer, showed Mrs. Dole to be very good at "wheeling and dealing." He explained that she neutralized opposition to her privatization bill by handing out hundreds of millions of dollars in DOT highway and bridge project funds to the districts of her opponents. Paul S. Sarbanes, a Democrat from Maryland and leader of a Senate filibuster against the bill, dropped his opposition after Mrs. Dole promised $72 million in improvement funds for Baltimore Washington International Airport. For Senator Ernest F. Hollings, a Democrat from South Carolina, tens of millions of dollars of highway bridge funds for his home district held sway.

"She was very effective, in a legislative sense, at doling out pork," said another Capitol Hill staffer.

The bill passed and the two airports were transferred to a regional authority.

Mrs. Dole had less success with another privatization effort, the sale of the Consolidated Rail Corporation, or Conrail, to the private sector. Her backroom dealing, in fact, precipitated Congressional intervention.

The federally owned Conrail had required hundreds of millions in federal subsidies to gain solvency. Its sale was a high-stakes venture, involving not only tax money but the future of the entire rail transport system of the Northeast and Midwest. Also at stake was Mrs. Dole's political reputation. Her husband was once again a presidential prospect. Privatizing Conrail and stashing a billion-dollar cash payment into the U.S. treasury would have looked awfully good. But Mrs. Dole's strategy failed to consider the complexity of the Conrail issue, and it underestimated opposition to the plan.

From the start, there were two options available. Conrail could be sold to another railroad company, or it could be made independent, a stand-alone corporation, through a public offering of stock. Mrs. Dole, acting on railroad industry claims that Conrail could not survive as an independent company, chose the former course of action. After evaluating bids for the railroad, she decided to sell the government's 85-percent share in Conrail to Norfolk Southern for $1.2 billion.

There were a host of problems associated with her decision, including charges that the proposed sale, the largest railroad merger in U.S. history, would be anti-competitive. *Traffic World*'s Don Byrne, who covered the Conrail saga for 13 years, called it a "real sweetheart deal." He explained, "She was not aware of what she was doing to the railroad system in this country. She didn't have a clue. The Norfolk deal would have eliminated competition from Maine to Florida. It also would have cheated the public out of a huge amount of money."

"That railroad belonged to the people. They had paid for it. She was determined to give it away. And it almost happened, that's the scary part," Byrne said.

Under Mrs. Dole's plan, Norfolk would have inherited Conrail's back tax credits. Consequently, the Congressional Budget Office estimated the purchase would cost Norfolk just $200 million, not $1.2 billion, which had already been a below-cost figure; analysts had pegged Conrail's worth at $2 billion. For $200 million, Norfolk

Southern stood to gain a monopoly on the entire East Coast and parts of the Midwest railroad system.

The battle over Conrail got nasty. Congressman John Dingell, Chair of the House Energy and Commerce Committee, announced an investigation and charged the Reagan Justice Department with destroying key documents regarding anticompetitive aspects of the sale. The charms of the woman who was nicknamed "Sugar Lips" on Capitol Hill did not work on the powerful Michigan congressman. While Mrs. Dole attributed Norfolk Southern's withdrawal of its bid for Conrail to changes in the tax law, in reality, Dingell's staunch opposition killed the deal. She was forced to abandon the proposal and open a public offering of Conrail stock, a move she had adamantly opposed.

Mrs. Dole lauded the sale of Conrail as a major victory of her administration, the "flagship of privatization." In reality, it was a stunning political defeat for the secretary.

Increasingly, Mrs. Dole found herself under attack. *Air Transport World* characterized DOT under Mrs. Dole as the "worst offender in the grandstanding sweepstakes," and called her and a deputy "opportunists." *Traffic World* described her response to air safety as "a carefully orchestrated public relations dog-and-pony show constructed to allay public fears, not remedy the situation," and said it was time for her to get out. The Aircraft Owners and Pilots Association also called for her resignation.

Mrs. Dole did resign, effective October 1, 1987. Ralph Nader told the *Washington Monthly,* "She comes in as a consumer advocate and misuses her reputation to avoid criticism." Her administration, he said, was "an epidemic of lost opportunities and surrendered authority." Congressman Norman Mineta was "disappointed with her ability to follow through on her rhetoric with concerted actions." Congressman Guy V. Molinari of New York observed, "I don't think Mrs. Dole can leave with a sense that she has made a contribution to improving the safety and efficiency of air transport in the country. Service has declined. We have seen just minimal increases in controller staffing. There have been increases in near collisions. She is very good at public relations. She is a very bright lady."

Fellow southerner Senator Wendell H. Ford was more charitable. He described Mrs. Dole as "dedicated and tireless," having done "an excellent job in the context of an administration that has been difficult to persuade on a number of transportation safety issues."

President Reagan accepted Mrs. Dole's resignation, saying, "the reason behind it will strike a chord with everyone who values the very human emotions that underlie public life at its finest."

Glamour magazine took a different view: "From Elizabeth Dole, who quit her Cabinet post, we learned that some women will still ride in the back of the bus if they think it will take them to the White House."

Once again, Mrs. Dole was on the campaign trail for her husband. And, once again she earned rave reviews. Syndicated columnist Mary McGrory called her a "dream campaigner." The *Chicago Tribune* dubbed her "radiant as a movie star, as regal as a queen," and remarked that her personal style of campaigning made each person she met feel "special."

Unlike Dole's ill-fated 1980 campaign, the 1988 race for the nomination brought up thorny questions about the finances of both the senator and his wife. The Doles' relationship with Duane Andreas, the CEO of Archer Daniels Midland (ADM), a $4 billion grain and commodities company based in Decatur, Illinois was a particular controversy. Bob Dole, the ethanol industry's leading advocate on Capitol Hill, had successfully opposed President Reagan's attempt to eliminate federal subsidies for the fuel, a boon for ADM. He denied that he had done favors for ADM, maintaining that his ethanol advocacy benefited his Kansas constituency. The Doles purchased a condominium from Duane Andreas at well below market value. Senator Dole stated that the condominium was his wife's property and that he had no knowledge of the real estate purchase. The deed for the property listed Mrs. Dole and her brother John as owners.

In 1980, Mrs. Dole loaned $50,000 to her husband's financially strapped presidential campaign. Questions about the legality of this transaction had been raised in 1980, when the Federal Elections Commission (FEC) investigated the loan. The senator told FEC investigators that his wife's assets were jointly held. The FEC took no action, however, citing ambiguity in Kansas's community property law. During the 1988 campaign, when the issue revived, the FEC claimed that it had lost internal documents relating to the case.

Days before the Iowa caucuses, yet more allegations surfaced. Charges of improprieties again arose concerning the awarding of a $26 million government contract to another former Dole aide, John Palmer. Palmer's company, EDP, won a lucrative contract to manage food service operations at an Army base in Missouri. Yet EDP's experience in food service management was minimal. The Bush campaign asked the House Small Business Committee to investigate the matter. The committee found that criminal laws might have been broken in the awarding of the contract; Dole aides had improperly applied pressure to win the Army contract for Palmer. Committee chairman John J. LaFalce of New York said the contract award was "replete with appearance of improper actions." But he had "found nothing that suggests any U.S. senator was personally involved in any questionable event or occurrence." The committee referred the investigative file to the Justice Department for possible criminal action. Dole's subsequent withdrawal from the presidential campaign dissipated further action.

Despite the enmity that had developed between Bush and Dole during the primaries, by the summer of 1988, Mrs. Dole was vigorously campaigning for Bush. In November 1988, one month after *Ladies' Home Journal* named Elizabeth Dole one of "America's 100 Most Important Women," the Bush/Quayle team won the election. Mrs. Dole's name was once again bandied about for a number of high-level posts, including ambassador to the United Nations. She was instead nominated by President Bush as Secretary of the Department of Labor.

Mrs. Dole, then 52, told the President-elect, "Let me think about it, because I've got to see if I feel a sense of mission. I need to know more about the Labor Department." On seeing the material Bush's office faxed to her, Mrs. Dole concluded, "My word, it is the people's department."

Elizabeth Dole agreed to take charge of the 18,500 employees and $31 billion budget of the Department of Labor (DOL). She was easily confirmed.

Bush maintained that the nomination "stood on its merits," but the appointment was viewed by many as an appeasement to Bob Dole. Frank Swoboda, DOL reporter for the *Washington Post,* called Mrs. Dole's DOL appointment "the Bush payoff." Swoboda's observation was based on Mrs. Dole's installing aides from her husband's campaign at the department. She brought with her from DOT her chief of staff, Robert Davis, whom she named solicitor. Jenna Dorn was made assistant secretary for policy, DOL's top research slot. Joining her Labor coterie from the Bob Dole political camp was attorney Roderick DeArment, who had been chief of staff to Senator Dole. DeArment was named deputy secretary of labor. Dale Triber Tate, former deputy press secretary and campaign spokeswoman for Senator Dole, became assistant secretary for public and intergovernmental affairs. Kathleen Harrington, director of Elizabeth Dole's office during the 1988 "Dole for President" campaign, was appointed assistant secretary for congressional affairs.

Rounding out Mrs. Dole's team was John Heubusch, former chief of staff to Congressman Denny Smith, a conservative Republican whose office also employed Kurt Pfotenhauer, Jenna Dorn's husband. Heubusch was installed as Mrs. Dole's chief of staff. He, too, would become one of her loyalists.

Mrs. Dole's tenure at the Labor Department was brief, her record mixed. There were accomplishments, such as the improved enforcement of workplace safety standards by the Occupational Safety and Health Administration (OSHA), and a risky intervention in the Pittston coal strikes, which prompted an eventual settlement. She was also credited with launching initiatives to increase job training for youths and to crack down on employee pension fund fraud.

But there were serious shortcomings in Mrs. Dole's management. While she spoke of the rights of women and minorities, child labor abuses, worker safety, worker training, and minimum wage, little of what she said led to permanent changes in government policy. And her actions often contradicted her words. As director of the Office of Public Liaison under Reagan, Elizabeth Dole had been successful in keeping women, minority, and labor constituency groups at bay. Under Bush, she built superficial bridges with Labor. "She has done a pretty good job of keeping the unions off the President's back by keeping an open door with them while at the same time not giving them a whole lot," Paul Weyrich, a prominent "New Right" Republican, told the *National Journal.*

Dole press secretary Dale Tate credited her as the architect of the White House strategy to fight labor's efforts to increase the minimum wage and bottle up much of the rest of the union agenda, including issues like family leave. In the end, the minimum wage was raised, but not as high as labor and Democrats in Congress wanted. Similarly, when the issue of parental leave came before the Congress, Mrs. Dole—who had pledged to fight for working families as Secretary of Labor—said she would recommend a presidential veto. "I'm very much for parental leave," she announced, "but not in mandated form."

In February 1990, in response to congressional criticism about inadequate enforcement of child labor laws, Mrs. Dole held a well-covered news conference to announce "immediate action to step up enforcement" of child labor laws. "The children of America are our future," she said. "The Department of Labor will do everything in its power to protect children against those who violate our child labor laws." Two Department of Labor "strike forces" were dispatched in an unannounced sweep of thousands of businesses allegedly violating child labor laws. Reporters were invited to accompany investigators on the trail. At the conclusion of the sweeps, Mrs. Dole announced that inspectors had found 7,000 children working under illegal conditions. She pledged tough fines for violators.

Mrs. Dole's child labor "crackdown" came less than 24 hours before a House subcommittee was scheduled to begin hearings critical of DOL's enforcement of child labor law. Democratic Congressman Don J. Pease of Ohio called Mrs. Dole's child labor initiative a "finger-in-the-dike approach." Democratic congressman Charles Schumer of New York said that the spotlight could do some good, "But I think you have to do more than that."

Workplace safety issues carried big political dividends. Polls showed that safety was a number-one priority for workers, even ahead of good pay. Following federal hearings in 1990 on workplace safety, during which bereaved mothers who had lost their sons in industrial accidents testified, Mrs. Dole boosted OSHA's budget, stepped up enforcement activities, and referred more cases for criminal prosecution.

As a Capitol Hill staffer remarked, "Whenever the wave of public opinion was about to crest, [Mrs. Dole] got on it and rode it as far as she could."

That summer, Mrs. Dole unveiled her "glass ceiling initiative." In a written statement, she explained the project: "I have made this issue my top priority. For me, it is a matter of fairness and equity, born out of personal experience." Businesses risked losing federal contracts if discriminatory practices were not rooted out. In one case, an aerospace engine parts manufacturer paid $3.5 million in back pay to women "who were steered into traditionally female jobs when they were hired."

On October 24, 1990, she resigned as Labor Secretary after less than two years on the job. The *Washington Post* wrote, "In her twenty-two months as Secretary of Labor, Dole received unanimously low grades for her impact on policy." White House officials and Mrs. Dole denied that she was frustrated by a lack of clout in the Bush administration.

Ironically, two years after Elizabeth Dole left the Department of

Labor, an Inspector General audit found her office had been "a burial ground" for politically sensitive cases involving government whistle-blowers and employment discrimination. Some sex and other discrimination cases had languished there for as long as ten years. According to the audit, Elizabeth Dole was among five Labor secretaries in the past decade who allowed such cases to linger the longest.

CHAPTER TEN

REMAKING THE WORLD
1991

American Red Cross blood is as safe as it's ever been.

Elizabeth Dole
President, The American Red Cross

Even before he took a blood sample, Dr. Frank Saulsbury knew Anthony Kirby had AIDS. The University of Virginia physician listened attentively as the boy's parents told him about their son's "strange illnesses." When he was nine months old, Anthony had suffered a type of soft tissue infection on his face. At eighteen months, he was infected with giardiasis, a parasite in the bowel and colon that caused projectile vomiting. At two, Anthony had had an ulcer of the cornea which had since recurred.

For the past two years, since he was five, the child had been experiencing extreme fatigue, unexplained low-grade fevers, and pains in his limbs. His speech would slur at times. A neurologist thought there was some sort of central nervous system abnormality. But a battery of blood tests, a CAT scan, an MRI, and a spinal tap were negative or inconclusive. A chest X ray showed a cloudiness in his lung. At the suggestion of their doctor, the Kirbys sought the advice of specialists at the University of Virginia.

The first question Saulsbury asked during the Kirbys' October 17, 1990 visit was whether Anthony had ever had a blood transfusion. He expected an affirmative answer.

"No," Connie Kirby said. "Anthony never had a blood transfusion."

Was she sure? Saulsbury asked.

"Absolutely."

To Saulsbury, Anthony's parents seemed to be average middle class people, not likely high-risk candidates for AIDS. Darrell Kirby was a sales manager, his wife a superviser at Sears telecatalogue. They were bright, aware, clearly devoted parents. Another son, Mathew, who was five years older than Anthony, was well.

Anthony was very personable and intelligent. His parents told Saulsbury that despite his illness, he never complained, that he was happy and always had a smile on his face. He loved to ride his bike and play baseball and had a special fondness for babies and younger children. But he especially enjoyed performing magic tricks. Anthony explained how he could put a pencil through a penny and a sword through a ring. He had lots of rope tricks, too. Anthony was carrying a Cabbage Patch doll. He told Dr. Saulsbury its name was Davis Edmonds. Saulsbury figured the doll was there for Anthony's emotional comfort. Children often carried with them familiar objects, particularly in times of upset, and this was certainly a difficult time.

Saulsbury probed the Kirbys for any further medical history. There was one thing, Darrell said. Early in the summer of 1983, when Anthony was about six weeks old, they had noticed that the top of his head did not have the soft spot characteristic of infants. They consulted a specialist at the Charleston Area Medical Center in West Virginia, where the Kirbys had lived before moving to Virginia. A surgeon at CAMC confirmed that the problem was "craniosynostosis," a premature closure of the soft spot in the skull.

It was then that Frank Saulsbury realized he had been asking the Kirbys the wrong question.

"Did Anthony have the surgery?" he asked.

Yes, the Kirbys said. It had been purely elective. They were told that Anthony would not suffer any mental impairment should they opt not to correct the condition. But his head might be slightly deformed. The Kirbys decided that "life was hard enough with a normal head," and decided on the corrective surgery.

"And there had been no blood transfusion during surgery?"

No. The Kirbys were absolutely certain. As a matter of fact, that summer they had become aware of the risk of AIDS through blood transfusion and specifically told the surgeon that they wanted to donate their own blood for Anthony's operation. They said they specifically wanted to avoid blood from the general population. But the surgeon had assured them that no blood would be needed. Even if a transfusion were medically indicated, he said, Anthony's own blood could be "reused" or "recycled." Based upon that reassurance, the Kirbys scheduled Anthony's surgery for August 23, 1983 at Charleston Area Medical Center.

The operation went well. No mention was made of any blood transfusion.

Saulsbury took a blood sample. When he went to place a bandaid over the puncture on Anthony's arm, the little boy held up his doll.

"Davis gets the bandaids," Anthony said.

Dr. Saulsbury put the bandaid on the doll's bald head. Based on Anthony's lethargy and fever, he decided to admit the boy to the hospital. When Anthony's HIV serum antibody test came back positive, a non-diagnostic open lung biopsy revealed AIDS-related lung disorders. Saulsbury was not surprised. The parents were shattered.

That was October 1990. In mid-January 1991, Saulsbury finally received a response to his earlier letters and calls to the Charleston Medical Center Blood Bank. The supervisor there told him that Anthony had indeed received a transfusion and that the donor had been diagnosed with AIDS. The packed red cells had been supplied by the Tri State region of the Red Cross, in Huntington, West Virginia.

Ironically, less than two months before Anthony's transfusion, Tri State Red Cross had gone out of its way to reassure the public about the safety of its blood. Tri State director Dr. Mabel Stevenson was quoted by the local *Herald Dispatch* in June 1983: "I think it [AIDS] has been blown out of proportion [and] the scientific basis for the fear of getting AIDS by receiving blood has not been fulfilled." She acknowledged that two cases of AIDS had been reported in West Virginia, but she wasn't sure where.

Most occurrences, Stevenson said, were "related to lifestyle practices," and its victims tended to live in large cities.

Stevenson went further in promoting the Red Cross party line. She sent letters to Tri State's hospital clients, assuring them that the Red Cross was taking steps to address the "potential risk of transfusion-associated AIDS," to wit, initiating educational programs and developing procedures for excluding blood donations from individuals in these high-risk groups. She informed hospitals that "the possible risk of transfusion-associated AIDS is on the order of one case per million patients transfused." One consequence of "the understandable but excessive concern for transfusion-associated AIDS" were requests by patients and their physicians to have blood donors selected from family members, friends, co-workers, and even newly formed private donor clubs. These "directed donations" were not any safer than blood available through community blood banks. As a result, "the American Red Cross Blood Services does not provide 'directed donations,' " Stevenson told hospital clients

The *Herald Dispatch* article made its way to Fred Katz at Red Cross headquarters. In a handwritten note to Dr. Gerald Sandler, Katz asked whether it was "timely [and] appropriate" to introduce the concept of "donation call-in for the high-risk donors [who] 'had to' donate."A donor at risk for AIDS who had felt obliged due to outside pressure to donate could subsequently call the center and instruct that his blood not be used. "Fred," Sandler wrote back, "If I felt that such persons transmitted AIDS, I would add on [a] gimmic [sic] to our to-the-point position. Since I'm not terribly concerned about such donations I wouldn't shake the quiet waters unless necessary."

Five years after Anthony's surgery, Red Cross Tri State had received a call from a local hospital. A patient who had undergone cardiac surgery had since developed AIDS. The man's only risk factor had been a blood transfusion. Tri State initiated a Look-Back on that case. It concluded that one unit of blood that patient had received had been donated by an individual who had subsequently tested HIV positive. The donor was a gay man. He had regularly given blood to Tri State: every seven weeks, in fact, for a period of two years. Anthony had received seventy cc's of one of those units, which had been separated into platelets, red cells, and plasma and further distributed. Cutter Labs had also purchased plasma from that unit for pooling with thousands of other units to produce antihemophiliac factor.

Saulsbury wondered when, if ever, the Red Cross would have informed Charleston Area Medical Center about Anthony Kirby. It had been over seven years since the boy's surgery. Earlier intervention might have helped ameliorate some of his symptoms. It certainly would have spared him years of having been a "human pincushion" during countless futile tests.

As 1991 began, Tri State's Look-Back was only one of the Red Cross's many problems. Morale at its blood centers nationwide was also in peril. Local pride, historically the backbone of the Red Cross service culture, had been pummeled by the Dingell hearings and a perceived lack of direction from headquarters. A confidential report, released internally in January by an oversight committee at the Red

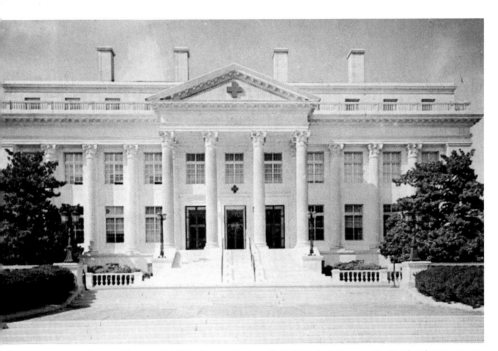

The American Red Cross National Headquarters Building in Washington, D.C. also known as the "Marble Palace". Along with two adjacent office buildings, this is the operating center for the worldwide services of the American Red Cross.

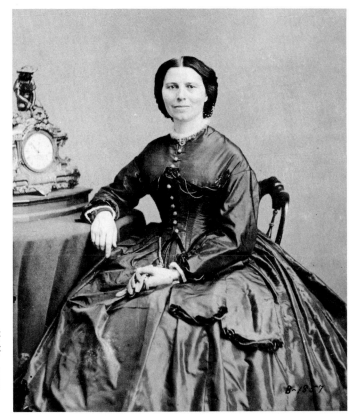

lara Barton was founder of ᴉe American Association of the Red Cross in 1881.
(*National Archives*)

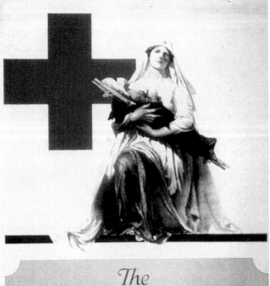

A World War I poster
advertisement for the
American Red Cross.
(*National Archives*)

In May of 1918, Red Cro
fundraisers sweep up mon
with a vacuum cleaner in fr
of the New York City Put
Library. (*National Archiv*

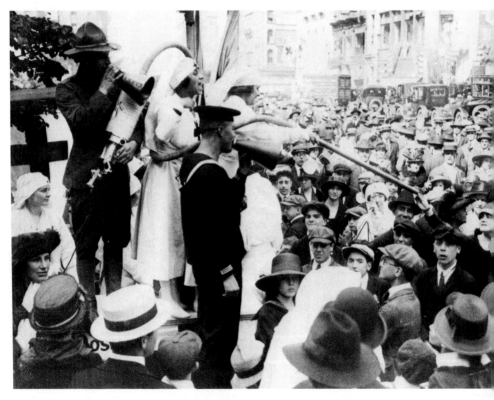

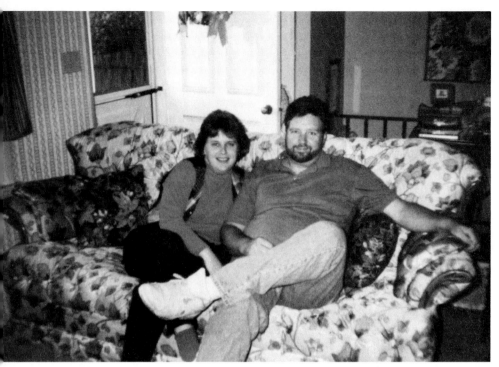

Janet and Roland Ray in 1996, thirteen years after he contracted transfusion AIDS.
(*Author Collection*)

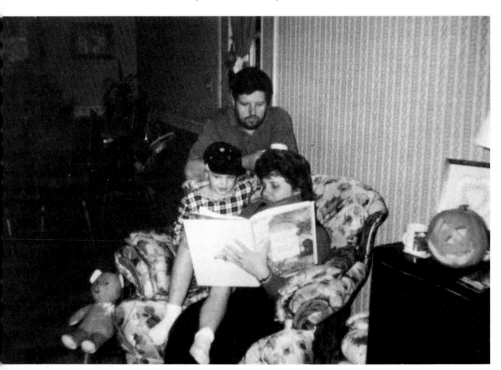

Janet and Roland Ray read to their daughter, Emily, who was born five years after her
father's HIV infected transfusion.   (*Author Collection*)

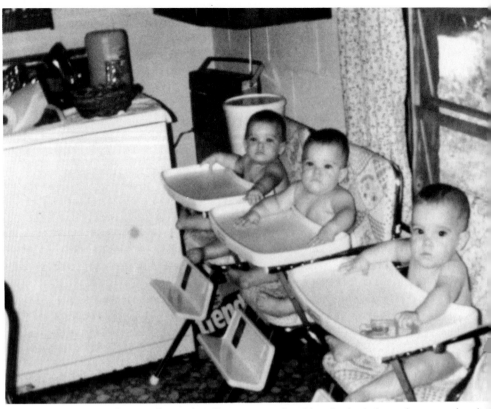

The triplets: Heather, Hailey and Holly at six months old in the highchairs their grandmother Jewelle Ann Michaels, gave them for their first Christmas. *(Courtesy of Jim Michaels)*

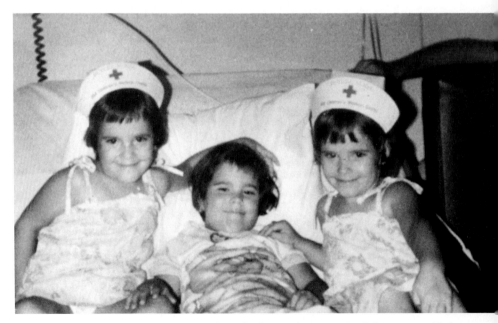

Hailey and Heather visit Holly in the hospital wearing Red Cross caps. Holly was hospitalized for a spleen removal. They were five years old. *(Courtesy of Jim Michaels)*

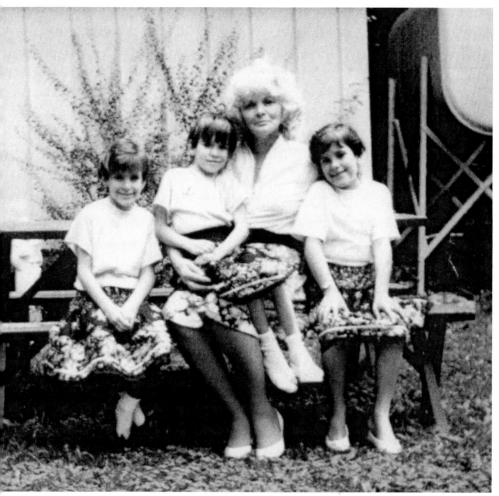

The triplets, age eight, with their grandmother. Hailey, Heather (*on Jewelle Ann's lap*), and Holly. Heather died of AIDS soon after this picture was taken.   (*Courtesy of Jim Michaels*)

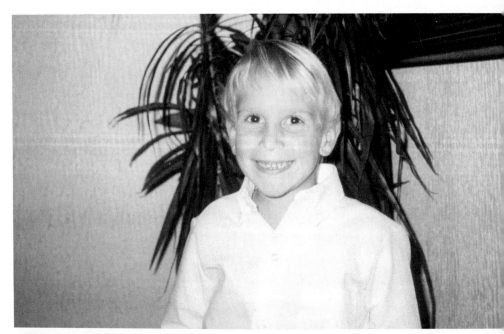

Anthony Kirby at seve
years old, just prior to h
diagnosis with HI
(*Courtesy of the Kirby Famil*

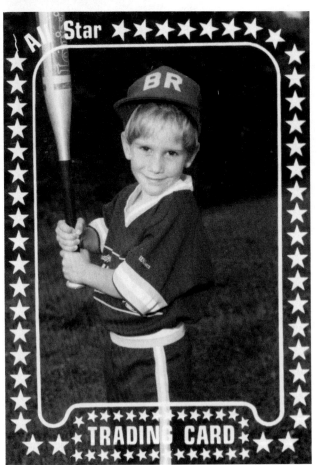

Anthony Kirby's All Star
Baseball Card for the
T-ball league, age six.
(*Courtesy of the Kirby Family*)

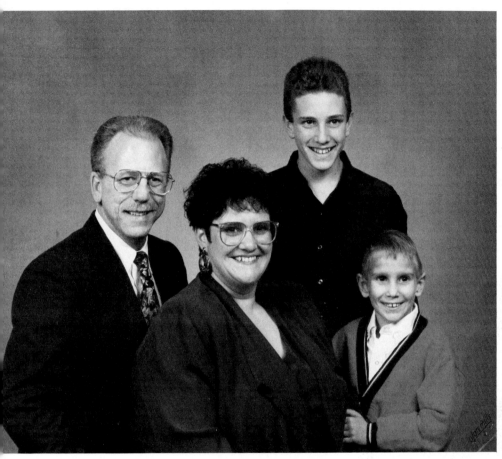

Anthony Kirby with his family; he is nine years old. (L–R) Darrell, Connie, Mathew and Anthony, the year he died. *(Courtesy of the Kirby Family)*

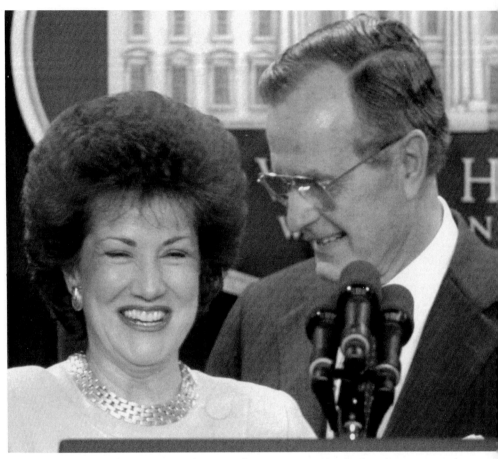

Introduced by George Bush on October 24, 1990, Elizabeth Dole announces her resignation from her cabinet post as Labor Secretary to head the American Red Cross. (*A/P Wide World Photo/Bob Daugherty*)

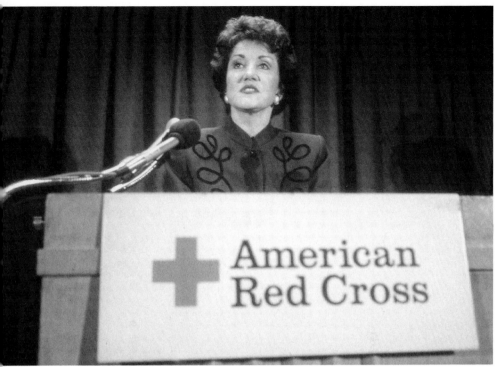

Elizabeth Dole, President of the American Red Cross.
(*Courtesy of James Colburn/Photoreporters, Inc.*)

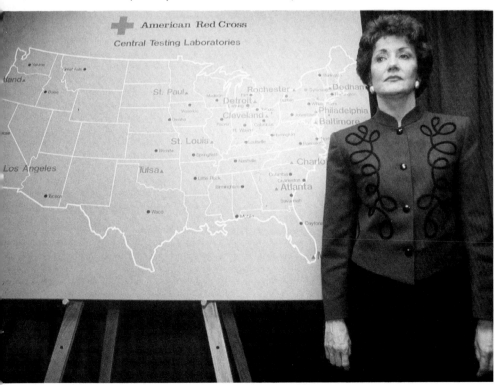

Elizabeth Dole anounces new testing of blood supply November 18, 1991.
(*Courtesy of James Colburn/Photoreporters, Inc.*)

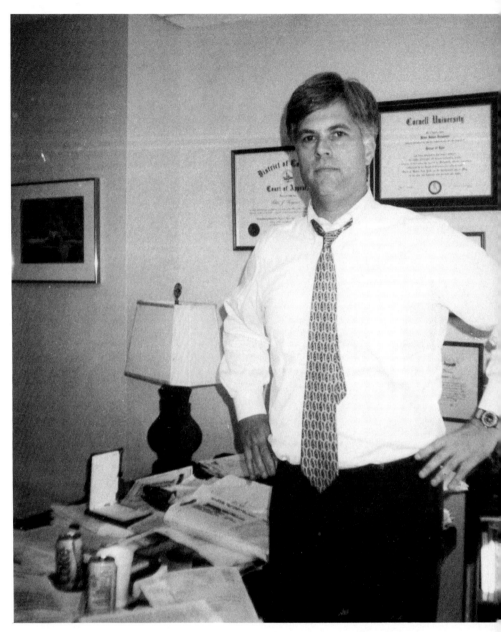

Peter Vangsnes, attorney, Ashcraft & Gerel   (*Author Collection*)

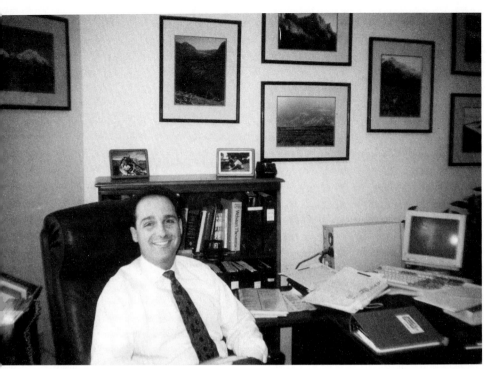

Chris Tisi, attorney,
Ashcraft & Gerel
(*Author Collection*)

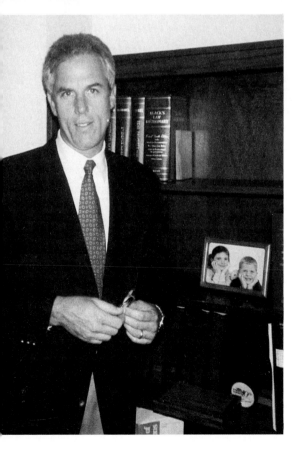

Michael Feldman, attorney,
Ashcraft & Gerel
(*Author Collection*)

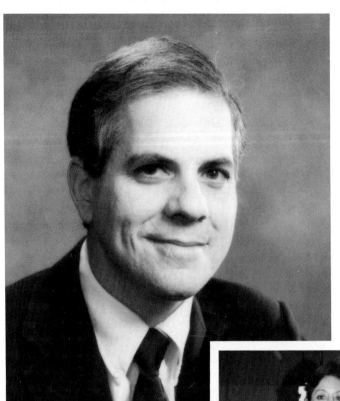

Dr. Edgar Engleman, director of the Stanford University Blood Bank.
(*Courtesy of Dr. Edgar Engleman*)

First Lady of Oklahoma, Cathy Keating presents Dr. Donald O. Gilcher (director of the Oklahoma Blood Institute) with an award for excellence in management of the institute during the aftermath of the Oklahoma City bombing. (*Courtesy of Oklahoma Blood Institute*)

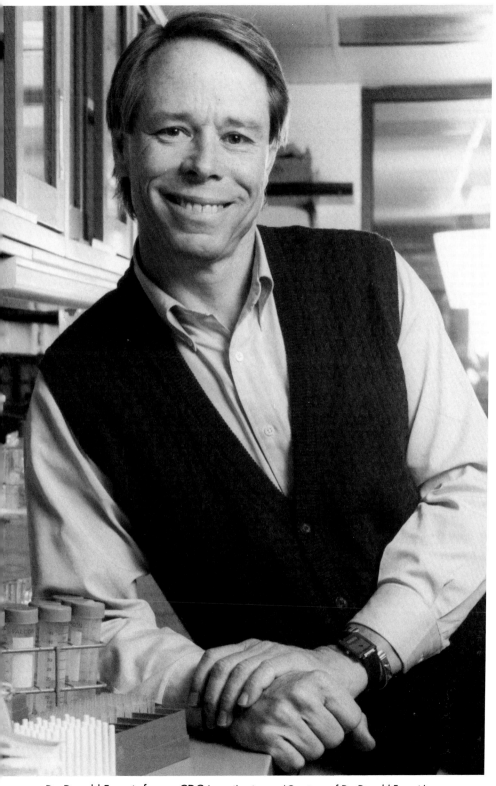

Dr. Donald Francis former CDC investigator.   (*Courtesy of Dr. Donald Francis*)

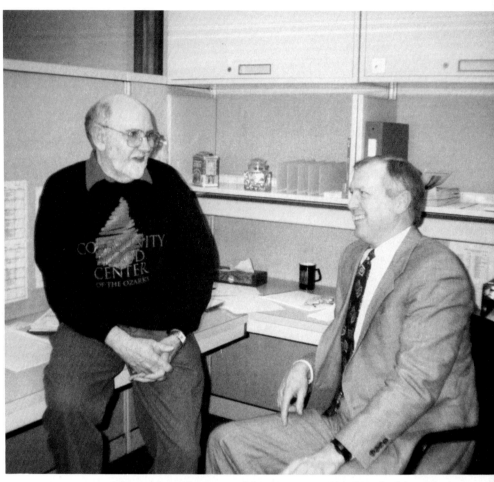

Gene Waite (left) and Don Thompson of the Community Blood Bank of the Ozarks. Waite and Thompson were among approximately one hundred Red Cross employees who resigned in protest from the Springfield, Missouri Red Cross Blood Center.
(*Author Collection*)

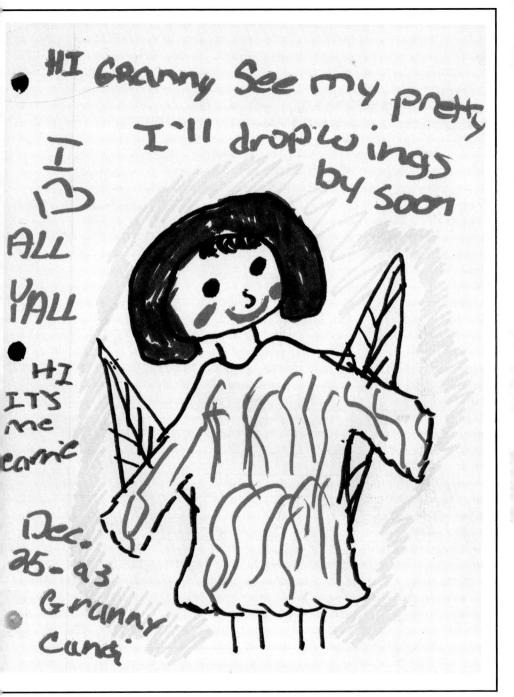

Drawing by Hailey Michaels, in 1991, of her sister Heather as an angel.
(*Courtesy of Jim Michaels*)

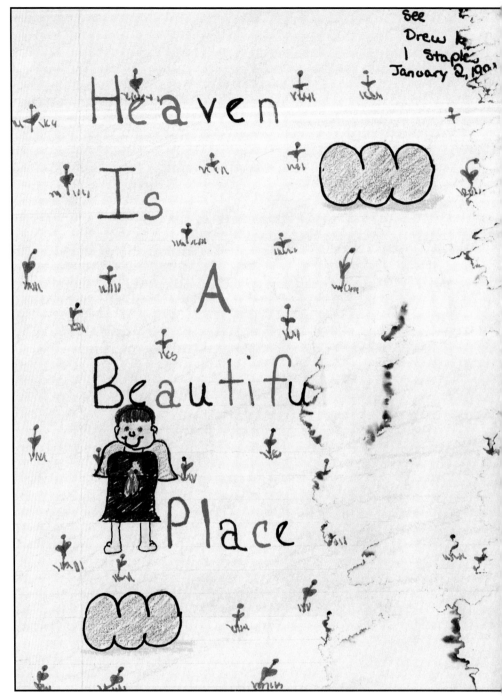

Drawing of Holly Michaels in 1994, after her sister Hailey's death from AIDS.
(*Courtesy of Jim Michaels*)

Cross, cited "mistrust and lack of accountability" as central problems. The committee advised attention and resources be refocused "from internal concerns to meeting the needs of customers and clients." It recommended a decentralization of authority, shifting power and money from headquarters to chapters. The goal was to eliminate the top heavy bureaucracy and streamline direct service delivery.

Enter Elizabeth Hanford Dole.

There was little doubt about Elizabeth Dole's ultimate political ambition. But as the eighties and yet another decade of Bob Dole's thwarted attempts at the White House came to a close, there was talk of Mrs. Dole herself seeking office. There was the possibility of a U.S. senate seat in her native North Carolina, or the governorship. There was speculation she might run as a vice presidential mate in 1996, or even try a future presidential bid.

Mrs. Dole said she had no plans for higher office. But she qualified that statement: "You never say 'never.' I've learned that in this town."

As a long-term survivor of Washington politics, Liddy Dole was a farsighted strategic planner who kept her fingers firmly on the pulse of public opinion as it played out in government and the press. Managing the nation's most revered charity would give her a high but benevolent profile and credentials comparable to that of a CEO of a billion-dollar corporation. Jack Andrews, an attorney who chaired the Department of Labor's Davis Bacon Appeals Board while Elizabeth Dole was Secretary of Labor, observed, "This is a lady who's been around a long time. Very smooth. She does not fall on her sword. She lands on the next lily pad."

The American Red Cross was the next lily pad.

Fifty-four-year-old Elizabeth Dole assumed presidency of the American Red Cross in January 1991, the year Blood Services marked it fiftieth anniversary. She told a standing room-only crowd in the Board of Governors Hall, "This is the first time I've been introduced as president of the Red Cross. It sounds good to me. I'm confident that you and I are a good match, united in a common mission to make a positive difference."

That mission: to ensure the public's health and safety. "There can be no higher trust than the blood of life we distribute," Mrs. Dole said. Just as she had stood in DOT's parking lot with a stop sign checking to see whether her employees were wearing seat belts, Mrs. Dole made as media-friendly a gesture of her allegiance to her Red Cross staff. Volunteers are, she told those gathered, "the heart and soul of American Red Cross. The best way I can let volunteers know of their importance is to be one of them—to earn the patch on my sleeve." She thus declined her first year's salary of $200,000. "I will be a volunteer," she said.

Mrs. Dole would earn, that year, $211,500 for eleven speaking engagements. She would donate a portion of that money to the Red Cross.

Mrs. Dole set out to create a tightly run ship. There would be little, if any, room for dissension. She chose her own management team as much for their loyalty as their competence. Most were recruited from among her coterie of followers during her years on Capitol Hill. Jennifer "Jenna" Dorn was named to the newly created position of Vice President for Policy and Planning. John Heubusch, who had been Mrs. Dole's chief of staff at Labor, was appointed vice president for communications. Michael Goldfarb, a colleague at DOT's Federal Aviation Administration, would be one of many of her high-priced consultants.

Longtime Dole loyalist Mari Maseng-Will would bring her savvy public relations skills to help hone Liddy Dole's latest image as powerful yet benevolent public servant. "She [Elizabeth] retained some of the grace and charm of the world she was brought up in," Maseng-Will told the *New York Times*. "I've often thought of her as a role model—how she carved out a role as a strong and effective woman, how she did not threaten people and could still be a leader." Maseng-Will, who was brought into and up through government by her "role model," would nonetheless warn her PR colleagues against bonding with their clients. At a Public Relations Society of America conference later that year, she explained, "The best thing you bring to the table is objectivity. Once you start seeing things through their eyes, you've lost your value to the client. (You) get pulled over the objective line."

Those at the Red Cross's highest level referred to this entourage as "Mrs. Dole's Special Team." "Elizabeth had this group, this entourage, which pretty much took care of her, pretty much surrounded her and kept her guarded," observed a former Red Cross Board member.

Jim MacPherson, head of CCBC, agreed. "When Mrs. Dole came to the Red Cross she wanted a budget that was her budget to bring in her own people. They advise her, they work only for her. They have no interest in the Red Cross at all, but the Red Cross pays for them. The Red Cross gave Elizabeth this huge consulting budget to do what she wanted. What she did do was bring a wonderful image to an organization in crisis."

Mrs. Dole told the public that the Red Cross would adhere to the same workplace standard she said she had sought at the Department of Labor. If employers failed to meet safety standards, they would have to "clean up [their] act or shut down." That philosophy translated at the Red Cross as, "All blood regions will meet or exceed [national standards] or they will not collect blood."

In early 1991, the Defense Department was gearing up for the Gulf War. In preparation for warfare, it was shoring up on blood; DOD asked the Red Cross to supplement its resources. Mrs. Dole had a far grander profile for the Red Cross in mind. With the help of the powerful PR firm Hill & Knowlton, a Gulf Crisis Fund was created. Its goal: to raise $30 million. It would be the largest wartime fundraising effort the Red Cross had undertaken since World War II, when it called for $50 million in contributions.

The fund's first, and most visible, contributor was Liddy Dole devotee President George Bush, whose $1000 check she brandished at a press conference. Her other former employer, President Ronald Reagan, volunteered as chairman of the campaign.

But it was in rallying her husband's longtime political patrons that Mrs. Dole proved her mettle.

Federal laws had set parameters on the influence corporate interests had over candidates; the ceiling on corporate gift-giving to political campaigns was $1000. However, corporate giving to private foundations and charities supported by their candidates of choice had long been accepted with a "wink and a nod." Such seemingly benign contributions enabled big business to show its gratitude for legislative favors or to accrue goodwill with elected officials. For industries which benefited from Bob Dole's politics, the Red Cross presented the ideal vehicle by which to say thanks.

One of the senator's most prolific supporters was among the first to show his goodwill to Elizabeth Dole's Red Cross. Archer Daniels Midland, the multibillion-dollar grain company run by longtime Dole pal Dwayne Andreas answered Mrs. Dole's Gulf War call with $500,000 channeled through its Andreas Foundation. It also put its corporate jet at her disposal. Previously, ADM had given nothing to the Red Cross.

According to the Center for Public Integrity, ADM was one of Bob Dole's "Top Ten Career Patrons." Ellen Miller, the director of another nonpartisan watchdog group, the Center for Responsive Politics, said of the Dole/Andreas relationship, "Bob Dole is a wholly owned subsidiary of ADM."

The Andreas family and company contributed more than $250,000 to Dole's campaign committees and foundations during his Senate and presidential campaigns.

Bob Dole had done well by Andreas. He had promoted legislation giving tax breaks to the ethanol industry, which was dominated by Andreas's company; ADM reaped $475 million in those tax benefits. Even Elizabeth Dole, who when she was the Secretary of Transportation had criticized the ethanol tax breaks as "inappropriate and contrary to the user-free principle." As senior member of the Senate Agriculture Subcommittee, Dole had not objected when USDA subsidies went to ADM, which profited to the tune of another $425 million. Dole had also sought tariffs on imports of ethanol, corn-based fuel, another economic boon for Archer Daniels, which derived nearly 40 percent of its earnings from corn sweeteners. A study by the Cato Institute, a libertarian group, disclosed that 43 percent of ADM's profits came from products that were subsidized directly or indirectly by taxpayers and government policy.

On a more personal level in 1982 the Doles purchased from Andreas an oceanfront condo in the Sea View complex in Bal Harbour, Florida. They paid $150,000, about 25 percent less than market price, on a delayed-purchase arrangement.

Yet another sudden Red Cross Gulf War contributor who profited from Bob Dole's tariff policies was the American Financial Corporation. A financial services company headed by Carl Lindner, AFC gave between $200,000 and $300,000 to the Red Cross's Gulf War Chest. Lindner had given hefty sums to both political parties over the years. The insurance conglomerate the American International Group, whose chairman, Maurice Greenberg, was a longtime Dole supporter, gave $500,000 to Mrs. Dole's Gulf War Chest through AIG's Starr Foundation; previously it had contributed only $1000 increments over three years to the Red Cross. AFC and AIG were among the companies which made their planes available to Elizabeth Dole.

Yet other Bob Dole supporters rallied for Mrs. Dole's cause, among them ConAgra, Federal Express (which would contract with the Red Cross as its exclusive overnight service provider), Forstman Little & Company, Morrison Knudsen Corporation, and the Alabama insurance firm Torchmark. Bob Dole contributor Marriott Corporation offered free accommodations to families visiting their soldier loved ones.

Within three weeks, Red Cross collected more than $7 million for its Gulf War Fund. By March, over $20 million had been raised. Mrs. Dole arrived in Kuwait bearing the Red Cross's first planeload of food—including baby formula, part of an initial $1 million relief package. She was photographed extensively stepping through rubble ("this is absolutely incredible. It makes your heart ache"), visiting hospital wards ("I want to urge people to help our troops and those left victimized by this war"), and consoling children ("It made you want to weep.").

But the Gulf War had also brought to the fore the Red Cross's own battles. In February, *60 Minutes* ran its story on Red Cross blood. The segment featured transfusion-AIDS victims, including Roland Ray.

Roland and Janet had been anxiously awaiting the news story. It had been delayed by the advent of the Gulf War, on which the media was focused. Janet hoped that the show would boost her husband's spirits. Roland's T-cell count had been fluctuating, and he had begun AZT. The drug weakened him and made him vomit. But there was something more, something internal that she felt had been failing her husband.

When they learned in 1989 that he was HIV positive, Janet's first thought was that she hoped she was, too, so she could go with him. But then there was Emily, and the fear that the baby might have been infected. Those anxieties overwhelmed Janet's anticipated loss of her husband.

And then there was the sickening realization that at some point, in some vague and not-so-distinct future, they would have to tell Emily.

As much as Janet wanted the *60 Minutes* story to air, she was afraid. They had told no one except their immediate family about Roland's AIDS. She had to admit she was afraid of going public. She knew about people's prejudices. She and Roland had been among those who had joked about AIDS. They, too, had been ignorant. But how would Wayne's and Sandra's peers react? Children could be so cruel.

Janet had been brought up a Catholic. She had always had a profound inner strength. That helped her live day to day with the anger, the fears, and the questions for which there were no answers. Some days, though, she felt she could not control her rage. When she and

Roland watched the Red Cross TV ads for Gulf War relief, Janet thought, What about us? We are a disaster the Red Cross caused. Where are they now?

CBS reporter Meredith Viera told viewers that Roland Ray was one of the victims of the D.C. region who had, at least, been notified. "According to FDA," Viera reported, "Red Cross neglected to inform hundreds of people they might be infected with the AIDS virus. A former Red Cross official told the FDA that tracking down victims is time consuming and expensive, and the Red Cross wanted to keep its budget down."

Holly LaLonde, a young woman who had had a transfusion in 1984 at Mount Carmel Hospital in Columbus, Ohio, had also received HIV-infected Red Cross blood. In anticipation of her elective surgery, she had donated one unit of her own blood. During surgery she had needed two units. It was the second unit that was HIV contaminated. LaLonde told CBS, "I think now they're trying to hide under a blanket of, 'But we're the Red Cross. We help people. How can you be mad at us?' And that's no good. You have to be accountable for your actions." Like Ray, LaLonde had initiated a lawsuit against the Red Cross.

But the Red Cross's problems were even more current, Viera explained. In 1991, its employees cited "working conditions [that] were so bad, and the pay so poor, that the turnover rate of technicians was 50 percent a year." Many of the 50 health care professionals and Red Cross employees *60 Minutes* interviewed "refused to tell us their stories on camera." "The Red Cross is such a powerful institution that they could be blackballed from ever working in the blood industry again."

Red Cross senior vice president Jeffrey McCullough assured viewers, "If I think the Red Cross cannot operate a safe and effective blood program that the public deserves, I will recommend to the Board of Governors that the Red Cross get out of the blood program."

If he had to make that decision today, based on FDA's investigation, would he recommend the Red Cross get out of the business of blood? Viera asked.

"Not at all," McCullough said.

When asked whether the military was concerned about the Red Cross's blood safety, Colonel Anthony Polk, director of the Armed Services Blood Program, said, "The short answer to that is no, because if we were, we wouldn't be accepting it."

After the show, Janet Ray was delighted and relieved at the community's reaction. Her friends called, sent lovely cards asking if there was anything they could do to help. The guys on Roland's construction crew who had often joked about gays and AIDS were humbled and supportive. And there were the calls and letters from strangers who had seen *60 Minutes.* With the exception of one or two, they were overwhelmingly reassuring. One family wrote just to say how touched they were by Roland's plight, others that they had sons, daughters, and husbands who had also contracted transfusion AIDS. One young woman called, crying. She told him she had been transfused in late 1982. Roland knew from his attorneys, Feldman and Tisi, that transfusion-AIDS cases in 1982 stood little chance in court. Roland stayed on the phone with her a long time. All he could do was listen, try to comfort her, and in so doing, comfort himself.

Several weeks later, another letter arrived. It was addressed "To the Man in Damascus, Maryland, who has AIDS." The writer told him that she, too, had a family member who had contracted AIDS during surgery. She was just writing to say he, Roland, was not alone, and that she had added him to her prayers.

Congressman John Dingell had promised a follow-up to his 1990 subcommittee hearings on the Red Cross blood supply. The new hearings were scheduled for April 18, 1991. For Red Cross the timing would be unfortunate. On April 17, the FDA informed the Northwest region in Portland, Oregon, that it intended to revoke its license for continuing to issue contaminated blood.

FDA had documented 51 violations of blood safety laws at the Pacific Northwest center as of March 1991. There were "approximately 350 discrepancies" in Portland's computer database, which resulted in a failure to defer high-risk donors whose blood posed a danger to recipients. FDA's random review of 20 of those discrepancies revealed that "unsuitable blood products had been released from three donors."

In addition, 594 donors had been entered into the Portland computer system with no social security number, essential for identifying donors. Since August 1990, when that problem had been identified, the FDA found "no attempt to investigate or correct these records."

Among the victims of Portland's blood was a sixty-year-old carpenter, Robert Jones. A Montana resident. Jones was visiting his son in Portland in late 1989 when he required emergency surgery. Four months later, he was told by the director of the Portland center that the donor, a married man who had frequented a prostitute, had AIDS. A month later, Jones tested HIV positive. "I never thought I could get AIDS, that only drug addicts and homosexuals got it," he told the press. "They told me and my family that the blood supply was safe and not to worry." Like Ray, who had received bad blood in Maryland, and LaLonde, who was a victim in Ohio, Jones, also, was suing the Red Cross.

John Dingell prefaced his April 1991 subcommittee hearings with a scathing indictment of the Red Cross. The organization's violations and its seeming disregard of congressional and FDA mandate were so overt that, Dingell told his colleagues, "It is now clear that the Voluntary Agreement may not have been fully complied with, and may not be an adequate mechanism to assure us of the safety of the blood supply. It now appears that the FDA will have to decide, and promptly so, whether injunction or other formal regulatory action is needed to protect the American public."

The Portland crisis particularly alarmed subcommittee member Ron Wyden. "If unsuitable blood products had been released from three donors at the Portland Center out of a test involving just twenty discrepancies," the Oregon Congressman said at the hearing, "certainly Northwest residents must be concerned about the possibility of other unsuitable blood products being released from the three hundred thirty other possible discrepancies."

Wyden had received a letter on April 8 from the director of the Pacific Northwest region, Dr. Frans Peetom. Dr. Peetom had assured Wyden that FDA's inspection showed that Portland was operating in Peetom's words with "excellent professional quality." At the hearings, Wyden asked Red Cross vice president Jeffrey McCullough, "Shouldn't Dr. Peetom retract this letter today?"

"No, I don't think so," McCullough replied. There had been, he pointed out, no recall issued.

"But Dr. McCullough, you just told Chairman Dingell just a second ago that in three hundred thirty instances you could not confirm that the blood was safe, and it had been unsuitably released, and yet you seem to want to stand by the letter that says that there is no question about the safety of those products."

McCullough said, "We had no evidence that anybody received infected blood."

"Isn't one of the reasons you have no evidence is that you were unable to perform confirmatory tests?" Wyden asked.

McCullough admitted that testing was "not accurate." He could not, he told the subcommittee, make an "absolute guarantee" that infected units had never been released in Portland. "I would say the testing system is not being carried out with the degree of tightness and the demand for meticulous attention that I expect this system to have."

When asked about the computerized donor deferral system which Red Cross promised a year before, McCullough insisted that a "new state of the art registry will be in operation in eighteen months." In the interim the centers would have to use existing systems.

"Pardon me if I express my frustration," Ohio Congressman Dennis Eckart said. "In 1988, the Red Cross and the FDA signed a Voluntary Agreement, one of the pieces of which was to create an appropriate technology-driven deferral donor system. There is not a consumer in America who has not experienced the problem of what happens when you buy something new. What's the curve going to look like if you get performance up to your optimal standards in September 1991, and then institute a new system? You will then have to go through the whole plethora of problems that will exist in introducing something that will be even more technologically driven than the current system, which you clearly have not been able to put in the field in an efficacious way to date."

The FDA had also informed the Red Cross's South Carolina region of its intent to revoke its license for serious safety problems, including mislabeling blood by type, a potentially fatal mistake. Like other Red Cross centers nationwide, South Carolina was in violation of not only the 1988 Voluntary Agreement, but Red Cross's own standard procedures. Problems caused by erroneously releasing blood, accepting unsuitable donors, and/or overall safety system failures also plagued St. Paul; Omaha, Nebraska; Farmington, Connecticut; the Greater Chesapeake and Potomac region; Wichita, Kansas; and Toledo. In Syracuse, New York, a delay in deferring at least sixteen donors who had tested repeatedly reactive for HIV and hepatitis resulted in the release of that blood for "routine transfusion" and manufacture into at least sixty-four blood components.

Some of the most egregious violators of the voluntary agreement, as well as the Red Cross's own standard safety procedures, were Omaha, Rochester, St. Paul, Penn-Jersey, Central Texas, Madison,

Tulsa, Huntington, West Virginia, Boise, Buffalo, Miami, and Albany, where nine erroneously released units had been made into injectable products. Patient deaths allegedly connected to contaminated blood in Appalachia and the Missouri-Illinois region had not been investigated. Missouri-Illinois Look-Back encumbered by shoddy recordkeeping that resulted in 1,400 discrepant records. At the Melville, New York center, thirty-seven units of mislabeled blood were issued to hospitals. Despite prior warnings about Abbott HIV tests, Melville had still not retested its inventory to assure safety.

In South Carolina, which was under FDA notice of license revocation, employees were not properly screening blood or donors and there was no indication of supervisory review. South Florida was not providing data to the National Donor Deferral Registry and it was not screening donors against that registry. As of July, at least thirty-seven regions were unable to comply with computerized production requirement because they had not installed a compatible system.

"No single license holder for blood has had the problems of the Red Cross," pointed out Dr. Gerald Quinnan, Jr., acting dean of the FDA's Center for Biological Evaluation and Research.

Mary Carden, the FDA senior investigator who had been commended at Dingell's 1990 subcommittee hearings for her diligence now reported, "I've seen important changes, but I haven't seen them made to the point where they've filtered down to the regions to ensure they stop unsuitable blood products from going out the door."

At the close of the session, John Dingell was not convinced that Jeff McCullough "or anyone in the Red Cross can successfully reform the blood program."

With the threat of federal injunction hanging over the organization she had promised to take in hand, Elizabeth Dole swung into action. She returned from Kuwait and convened a meeting of her top advisers. She would describe the outcome as "the most ambitious project the Red Cross has ever undertaken, the total Transformation of how we collect, process, and deliver half of the nation's blood supplies."

In a move similar to her other eleventh hour maneuvers made at the heels of regulatory mandates, Mrs. Dole announced a "remaking of the world of the American Red Cross." At the annual Red Cross meeting in San Diego on May 19, Mrs. Dole announced a $120 million "Transformation" program which would "revolutionize blood banking. Rather than just meeting standards, we will raise them. Instead of just fixing problems, we will spend our time preventing them."

Central to Transformation was a fundamental change in the Red Cross's longstanding public service culture. Transformation would entail "shifting to a pharmaceutical manufacturing atmosphere and style," a commodity-based approach to blood. Centralization of authority was key to putting into place a "tightly controlled environment where quality control is a top priority."

Mrs. Dole's "five-point plan" dictated massive changes in laboratory testing; donor recruitment, evaluation and deferral; blood collection and preparation; product management; and hospital and patient services. Step one, the centerpiece of Transformation, was a rotational center-by-center shutdown of each blood region for a period of eight weeks, to put into effect new safety procedures. During those rotational closures, the Red Cross's blood transport system would mobilize so that "not a single patient will go without the transfusion he or she needs."

Step two was a consolidation of the fifty-two blood centers' test labs into fewer than ten regional labs under the direction and control of headquarters. More internal inspections were promised.

The 1988 voluntary agreement had required the Red Cross to standardize its procedures. But despite "major efforts during the past six months," Mrs. Dole contended, the "variety of computer systems makes this impossible." Of the twenty computer systems, only four were certified. Red Cross "experts" at headquarters would, she said, evaluate the existing systems and a consulting firm would "structure and drive the process."

In addition, there would be a "state-of-the-art donor deferral registry [to] guarantee that healthy blood donors contribute to our system."

Lastly, the Red Cross's new president intended to create a regional Biomedical Board of Directors to work with Blood Services staff, ensuring "the adequacy and safety of the blood supply in each community."

"American Red Cross blood is the safest in the world," Mrs. Dole said, "but the key here is that we're going to make it as safe as it can be made, or we're not going to collect blood."

Many in the blood industry were stunned at Mrs. Dole's plan to shut down centers for two-month periods. Charles Mosher, the former chief operating officer and chief financial officer for Vermont/New Hampshire Red Cross, recalled, "You can't do that.

Whether she [Dole] didn't understand or was just trying to grab everybody's attention, everyone was just incredulous."

Mosher had left the Red Cross in the mid-1980s to form the Rhode Island Blood Center. An independent blood bank, Rhode Island maintained an amiable product-share relationship with the Red Cross. Unlike other industries, which could endure temporary shutdown, the blood industry dealt in a perishable commodity. Its delivery had to be timely. "It sounded good," Mosher said of the Transformation plan. "Red Cross was saying, 'We're taking this seriously, we're shutting everything down,' but it was just not practical." He predicted chaos. In the fallout, the Red Cross could be hurtling the entire blood industry over the precipice.

Unlike some of his peers, who hoped that upheaval at the Red Cross would send hospital clients and donors their way, Mosher took a broader view. As blood bankers, they all were "in the same barrel of apples. Failure of the Red Cross system will send a strong message to the people of this nation that we are a profession of incompetents. Certainly if we're not capable of providing a safe blood supply or managing our business, it can't be very safe to be a donor, either. Any diminution of public support will propel us into blood shortages the likes of which we have never seen."

Jim MacPherson was as skeptical of Mrs. Dole's plan. MacPherson had served for nearly ten years in regulatory affairs at Red Cross headquarters. In 1986, he became executive director of the Council of Community Blood Centers. When he heard about Mrs. Dole's dramatic announcement, MacPherson immediately sensed a political move. "This was an idea thought up inside the Beltway," he later recalled. "It was clearly a political gesture meant to appease FDA, where the pressure was coming from. It wasn't based in reality. Mrs. Dole's Transformation plan showed she didn't know what she was talking about. She had no understanding of what blood banking was all about."

For one, shifting to a pharmaceutical structure made the regulators, not the donors or hospitals, the clients of the Red Cross. "The Red Cross focused its energies on pleasing the FDA, but it forgot what its core constituency is—the reason it exists—which is to serve communities," MacPherson said. Why didn't Red Cross simply shore up its local infrastructure, as its internal review had recommended? He hoped that when Transformation was "vetted against reality," it would itself be transformed into "something more workable."

If not, MacPherson expected things would start falling apart.

Local centers had already begun to revolt. Many key regional administrators had not been informed of Mrs. Dole's plan. Like the general public, they had heard about Transformation through the media. That made for rather awkward press relations. Dr. David Jenkins, then director of the Red Cross's Louisville, Kentucky blood center, was outraged. In his view, "across the board" overhaul was plain and simple bad management. Louisville did not need fixing. It had become so profitable it was exporting blood to other regions. "Customers and donors were happy with us and suddenly these people from headquarters are going to come in and tell us what to do? You use us as a model, not shut us down."

Jenkins anticipated a higher cost of doing business locally and a drop in morale. "Community blood banks are the heart and soul of Red Cross. You are part of a system, but there is only so much benefit in being part of a dysfunctional family."

Insiders privy to Mrs. Dole's management style said that public *image*, not public *service*, was the driving force behind Transformation. One high-level former Red Cross blood service executive, who asked for anonymity for fear of reprisals, said that Transformation's purpose was simply to "enhance and protect Elizabeth's image as savior, someone who has everything under control. The Transformation plan was a PR spectacular. She got Dingell, Congress, FDA off her back for a while. The maneuver was: 'Let's pull one out of our hats to divert public opinion and buy time.' It was strictly politically handling."

Other insiders said Transformation reflected the true allegiance of its real architects, Mrs. Dole's Special Team, whose mission was to keep watch over the public persona of Mrs. Dole.

If Transformation's intent was to hone Elizabeth Dole's image in the eyes of those ignorant of blood banking, the plan was an immediate success. Congressman John Dingell knew Liddy Dole's proclivity for grand plans, which, experience had shown, often needed profound reality checks. Still, he lauded Transformation as "worthy of very high praise. I want to particularly commend Mrs. Elizabeth Dole, president of the Red Cross, for the extraordinary vision and courage which she had brought to this undertaking."

Dr. Louis Sullivan, who succeeded Margaret Heckler as Secretary of the Department of Health and Human Services and, who, by title, was a Red Cross Board member, described Transformation as "an exceptional management step. This is evidence that the new leadership of the Red Cross takes the issue of blood safety very seriously and has the courage to face up to the problems they have had in the past."

Even Ann Landers, who had attacked the Red Cross's failed disaster relief programs, now sung Liddy Dole's praises.

Red Cross's future secured, Mrs. Dole resumed her high-profile Gulf War tour. At her return to D.C., she learned that the cornerstone of Transformation, center-by-center shutdown, was not feasible. In closed meetings with her key advisers, she was told that her plan was neither economically nor operationally possible. At very least, the cost per region would be $100,000, a hefty price for Red Cross's fifty-two centers. Serious blood shortages could also ensue. Hospital relationships could be permanently damaged.

At the time, the principal concern expressed was public perception. One high-ranking official recalled that one of the first questions discussed was whether it was necessary to tell anyone that center closures were not feasible. The public's perception of change was a significant issue for upper management, and so it was decided that the matter could remain strictly internal. Thus, within less than two months of announcing Transformation, its centerpiece was scrapped.

Ironically, the summer of 1991 marked the tenth anniversary of the first formal acknowledgment of the disease that would be known as AIDS. In June 1981, the Centers for Disease Control reported that a new immune disorder of unknown causes had affected five gay men in Los Angeles.

By summer 1991, low morale and interpersonal friction had begun to take its toll at headquarters. In July, senior vice president Jeff McCullough announced his resignation.

McCullough publicly stated that he wished to return to the University of Minnesota to continue his research. But many officials within the Red Cross cited strained relations between him and Elizabeth Dole. A former board member recalled, "She started getting into his business, where he believed she didn't belong, making decisions that were his to make." Another high-level officer remarked, "It was complete and absolute warfare. He was ready to throttle her. It was all about control with her."

As Red Cross vice president Dr. William Miller saw it, Dr. McCullough and Mrs. Dole "couldn't come to terms."

Dr. McCullough declined to comment further.

Promises to the Dingell subcommittee and the public notwithstanding, Red Cross's system-wide operations remained as haphazard as ever. High-tech consultants wrangled unsuccessfully with various computer designs to fulfill Mrs. Dole's promise of a national, centralized computer system. Millions of dollars and many months later, there was still no centralized system. Nor were there procedures for training individuals responsible for reviewing error and accident reports, or for analysis of those reports for corrective action. There was, most significantly, no adequate procedure for reviewing and tracking suspected post-transfusion-HIV infection cases by headquarters. Meanwhile computer contracts continued to be renewed on a regional basis, generally with longtime vendors. One was veteran government contractor Unisys Corporation. In 1991, Unisys settled charges brought by the Department of Justice alleging its involvement in influence peddling; it paid the government $190 million. The following year, the Red Cross would award Unisys a $3.7-million-dollar contract to serve five regions.

The FDA continued through year end to document massive noncompliance with blood safety regulations. A July error report from the former D.C. region indicated there were approximately 4,500 donor history records missing for blood collected between 1986 and 1989. Those records were essential to HIV Look-Back investigations. Out of a total of 333 Look-Back cases, the FDA reviewed five at random. It found that eight plasma products from a donor who was implicated in an early 1980s transfusion-AIDS case had been released. Years later, no recall had yet been issued.

D.C. residents were particularly outraged when in December, the Red Cross announced it would tie up what it called "loose ends." It finally informed 300 donors to the former D.C. region that the blood they had given as long as six years earlier had shown indications of HIV reactivity. A Red Cross spokesperson explained that it did not inform "everyone who shows an initial positive result" to avoid them undue worry and stress.

Meanwhile, Elizabeth Dole continued to make Transformation promises. In October 1991 she announced an even more ambitious plan for computerization, one that would "go beyond" the original proposal. Hiring on yet more experts to assist in this development, she set 1994 as the new date for national implementation.

"Red Cross kept writing specs for what each system had to have, the lists got longer," vice president William Miller observed. "All those consultants, Arthur Anderson and Boston Consulting, threw up their hands. Money kept being spent. Everything was orchestrated to make her look good, put her in a jacket, and whisk her off to kiss Ethiopian babies, yet the fundamental issue with service was not being addressed."

It was, Miller said, "scandalous, the amount of money that got dumped into gross mismanagement."

On the Red Cross's 1991 tax return, Boston Consulting Group and Information Data Management each earned about $1.9 million. A revolving door of consultants—51 on the national level, 51 for other sectors—earned, in total, over $3 million. Consultants called in to help the Red Cross address government crack down made $9.5 million; a total of $50 million went toward expenses and salaries to address legislative issues.

By year end, Mrs. Dole had increased by $17 million the cost to implement Transformation; the new price: $137 million. That first year, Transformation added $113.5 million to Blood Service's budget, an 8-percent hike over fiscal 1990–1991.

There was no center-by-center metamorphosis, no viable blueprint for a centralized computer system, no local biomedical review board—only chaos, low morale, and big bills from pricey consultants.

Still the Red Cross ended 1991 with the distinction of being the second best funded and staffed charity in the U.S. Its $1.1 billion budget ranked just below that of YMCA's $1.3 billion, but above the United Nation's Development Program's $800 million. Its paid staff of 25,394 was topped only by the Salvation Army's legion of 38,549.

But to many, the Red Cross's honeymoon with Elizabeth Dole appeared to be over.

CHAPTER ELEVEN

BLOOD MONEY

1992

Integrity is our bottom line.

Norman Augustine
Chairman of the Board
The Red Cross

The ongoing international battle between the French and U.S. governments over patent rights to the AIDS test had once again thrown John Dingell's Subcommittee on Oversight and Investigations of the House Committee on Energy and Commerce into revisiting the issue of blood safety. Scientist Luc Montagnier of the Pasteur Institute claimed discovery of the virus that caused AIDS. The National Institutes of Health attributed HIV discovery to its own Robert Gallo. In mid-1985, the Pasteur Institute sued the NIH for breach of contract and patent rights. In March 1987, the two governments had negotiated an out-of-court political settlement, apportioning for AIDS test royalties.

Gallo retracted his discovery role, in part, in early 1990. Confronted with new genetic evidence, the NIH scientist was forced to concede that the Pasteur Institute had, in fact, discovered the HIV virus. Pasteur Institute was now demanding a renegotiation of royalty shares to reflect Gallo's admission. It was also asking for $20 million in patent earning reparations.

The dispute was more than an issue of appropriate credit. Dingell's subcommittee was examining whether the U.S. government, specifically the Department of Health and Human Services, had been remiss or possibly corrupt in driving Gallo's claims. Also implicated were the U.S. Department of Justice, which went to battle for Gallo, and the Patent Office.

The fracas over Gallo had prompted a series of articles in the *Chicago Tribune*. The subcommittee had been alerted, through that series and an NIH whistle-blower, to a tangential but just as serious issue: Red Cross's use of Abbott Laboratories AIDS test kits when the more reliable Genetic Systems test had been available.

It was in connection with the Abbott and Red Cross relationship that Dingell was now contacting Elizabeth Dole.

The congressman had learned that in May 1986, the Red Cross had been aware of problems with Abbott's test kits. Despite this knowledge, it had failed to take remedial action. In a January 16, 1992, letter to Mrs. Dole, John Dingell wrote that the Red Cross's inaction had resulted in the "strong possibility that HIV contaminated blood made its way into the United States blood supply."

John Dingell wanted to know how this had happened. When did Red Cross first learn of the problem of false negatives with Abbott's HIV blood test? What was its response? Why did the Red Cross permit the problematic test to remain in use for over eight months while Abbott attempted to remedy the defects? During that period, did the Red Cross alert potential recipients of its blood products of the possibility that they might receive HIV-contaminated blood? Had any recipients of Abbott-screened Red Cross blood sued?

Dingell sent a similar letter to Duane Burnham, chairman and CEO of Abbott Laboratories, also requesting pertinent documents regarding Abbott's correspondence with the Red Cross.

Dingell's subcommittee was already facing significant pressure from powerful supporters to lighten up its inquiry concerning Dr. Gallo. Bringing in two more formidable entities, the Red Cross and the $6.8 billion Abbott Labs, would further complicate the subcommittee's life.

In July 1991, Dr. Suzanne Hadley resigned as deputy director of NIH's Office of Scientific Integrity, where she had been chief investigator on the Gallo case. Hadley had led investigations into sensitive areas like scientific misconduct which implicated, in some cases, Nobel laureates. As such, she was used to flak from the "science politics" sector. But she was not prepared for the kind of ferocity surrounding Gallo.

In early 1991, Hadley had brought the question of Gallo's claim of HIV discovery to the attention of NIH director Bernadine Healy. The Office of Scientific Integrity had found that Gallo's report on his isolation of the AIDS virus contained numerous falsifications of data and misrepresentations of the methods used. In the OSI report, Hadley criticized Gallo for "an unhealthy disregard" for professional and scientific ethics.

Political pressure over her findings caused her to resign and she headed for John Dingell's subcommittee. The Gallo/NIH patent claim warranted, Hadley believed, congressional investigation.

Over the space of one weekend, she authored a report entitled "The Great AIDS Cover-up," which she submitted to Dingell. By August 1992, Hadley and two of Dingell's most aggressive staffers were on the trail of Gallo. That led them, in turn, to the Red Cross and Abbott Labs.

Dingell's "sweeping document demand" produced memos from the Red Cross, Abbott, and FDA, that surprised even Hadley. "I was shocked and disgusted," she later recalled. "That threesome—Red Cross, Abbott, and FDA—had an unhealthy, unholy relationship. They had this song and dance they played around each other. My greatest concern was with the FDA, because it is nominally the public servant. But with that said, the Red Cross is nominally a public interest organization. Even if it were negligence and bumbling, still it is extraordinary that the Red Cross kept its head in the sand for so long."

During a February 13, 1992 meeting with Red Cross in-house associate general counsel Edward Wolf, a former Arnold & Porter attorney, and Carol R. Byerly, the Red Cross government relations officer, Hadley and Dingell's investigators were told that many of the requested documents had been placed under court-ordered protective seal. Those protective orders related to a 1988 lawsuit Genetic Systems had filed against Abbott and the Red Cross. Genetic Systems sought to enjoin execution of the contract between Abbott and the Red Cross, alleging it constituted a monopoly. The court found that Genetic Systems did not prove its claim and denied the injunction.

In its response to Dingell's inquiry, the Red Cross defended its actions with Abbott. Despite years of documentation, including internal memos, meeting minutes, and its own comparative data on the Abbott and Genetic Systems tests, the Red Cross told Dingell that it had "acted responsibly and expeditiously to protect and enhance the safety of the nation's blood supply [and] strenuously disagree[d] with the contention that there was a period during which it was using a 'defective' test manufactured by Abbott." It also defended Abbott.

Abbott also denied culpability. It told Dingell, "Studies comparing the performance of one commercially available test to another did not establish that any one test was consistently superior to another."

There would be at least twenty transfusion-AIDS lawsuits, some filed as late as 1990, against Abbott and/or the Red Cross, citing faulty tests which had not been withdrawn from the market. The suits were brought nationwide, including in New York City (Lenox Hill Hospital), Houston (Veterans Administration Medical Center), Chicago, Charleston, and Walton Beach, Florida. Among the victims was a young mother in Philadelphia who claimed that her receipt of a transfusion of false-negative blood in December 1988 would subsequently infect her two infants with AIDS.

"Frankly," Hadley said, "where it gets to be more despicable is when they [the Red Cross] attempted to defend that kind of behavior. Especially when you are a public interest organization, the thing to do is get out in front of this stuff and say, 'We screwed up; we are sorry. We wished we hadn't done that.' Instead, what they did was jump into litigation with both feet and settle these court suits in a way so that the public knows little or nothing about the outcome."

The Subcommittee on Oversight and Investigation would release its report in 1995. It found that the H9 cell line which Abbott used "had an inherent defect that made it particularly problematic. The defect had a significant deleterious impact on the HIV blood tests licensed under Gallo."

The report further found that government lawyers, concerned with protecting U.S. patent rights, had also been involved. The subcommittee's final report cited a number of tactics the government had been considering to keep Abbott on the market. These included suing Genetic Systems for infringement of Gallo's blood test patent, going so far as to threaten to withhold royalty payments to the Department of Health and Human Services unless HHS sued (it did not). The government attorneys were also contemplating disadvantaging Genetic Systems by stringent enforcement of import restrictions on the Pasteur Institute virus. And they were exploring illegal acts like "covertly intercepting and recording employees' conversations." Notes in one of the government attorney's files, labeled "Criminal Investigation," included copies of federal statues governing wiretaps and covert surveillance strategies and a handwritten note of caution: "Hot potato. High visibility case—have to be extremely careful with such."

Political pressures and shifts on Capitol Hill forced Dingell's committee to abandon further inquiry into the relationship between Abbott and the Red Cross.

As of March 1992, about one million Americans had been infected with the AIDS virus: between 12,000 and 15,000 had been infected through blood products; and 60 percent of the nation's 20,000 hemophiliacs had been contaminated. As to how many victims were suing, estimates ran into the several hundreds. By the end of 1992, Red Cross attorneys had succeeded in sealing between 7,000 and 8,000 "confidential" documents. The exact number was a closely guarded secret by the blood bank defendant. One California law firm alone was handling 70 transfusion-AIDS cases. Irwin Memorial Blood Bank in San Francisco was itself facing over 25 transfusion-AIDS lawsuits.

Infected hemophiliacs were contemplating a unified class action suit on behalf of as many as 9,000 victims.

Since Mrs. Dole had joined the Red Cross, the organization had begun spending millions of dollars fighting transfusion-AIDS victims in court. Its in-house legal department of thirteen, including seven lawyers, was supplemented by outside counsel, which was paid about $4 million to defend against, for the most part, transfusion-AIDS claims. But the Red Cross had other gripes that captured its legal attention, like the one in a Kentucky town by the name of Red Cross. The rural enclave had been founded in the late 1880s. Its 210-student public elementary school had borne the name Red Cross School since the early 1900s. But almost 90 years later, the American Red Cross came upon the perceived infraction. The billion-dollar organization informed the school's principal that the "use of the Red Cross name is considered unauthorized."

The Red Cross opted not to sue the Red Cross School. But it had 75 similar cases pending.

Until mid-1992, the Red Cross had avoided trial as a defendant in transfusion-AIDS cases. Courts were generally ruling in favor of its defense that it had conformed to the industry's customs and practices. But a few lawsuits against other blood banks had proceeded to trial; the outcome cost Red Cross's peers dearly. A Denver jury verdict in 1989 awarded $5.5 million to a woman who was transfused during childbirth on March 22, 1985. The hospital had received the new AIDS test kits nine days earlier, but had not used them on blood previously collected and stored. The woman had received such blood. In another childbirth transfusion suit, a Seattle, Washington jury awarded $1.8 million to the victim. That case was the first in which an implicated donor took the stand. It underscored the importance of learning the donor's identity, a disclosure routinely fought by the Red Cross. The donor who had given blood at least twenty times testified that he was gay. He told the jury that if the blood center had asked gay men to defer, he would have not given blood.

In two other non–Red Cross cases, a Kings County, Washington jury awarded $12 million to a transfusion-AIDS victim who sued Puget Sound Blood Center. And in Arizona, the largest state award: $28 million in a case of a 5-year-old Arizona boy who had been given an unnecessary transfusion; the blood was HIV infected.

The Red Cross and Children's Hospital in Los Angeles were named in another highpayout lawsuit. In this case a ten-year-old girl had contracted AIDS from a transfusion during open-heart surgery in June 1984. Her parents sued the blood supplier, the hospital, and her cardiac surgeons for failing to obtain informed consent and not conveying the risks of AIDS in blood transfusions. The Red Cross was accused of failing to institute surrogate testing and failing to warn the medical community and general public of the risks associated with transfusion. The suit also alleged negligence by the hospital in failing to postpone the procedure until the availability of an HIV blood test, which was imminent.

The hospital argued that had it complied with the prevailing standard of care in 1984. The Red Cross argued that the medical community was well aware of the risks of blood transfusion in 1984, and that surrogate testing was not the accepted standard of care. Days before the case went to trial, the Red Cross settled.

The jury decided against the hospital. It found the value of the girl's lost earnings to be $2,250,000, "based on evidence" that she had an IQ of 134 and wanted to be a physician. The court voided one of two $250,000 "pain and suffering" awards under California's statutory limit of $250,000 for noneconomic damages, reducing the total award from $3 million to $2.7 million.

The girl's attorney, Martin Berman, attributed the Red Cross's conciliation to its "being very nervous about the case." By June 1984, the HIV virus had been identified and many blood banks on the West Coast, including Red Cross's San Jose so-called "test site," had followed Stanford University Edgar Engleman's lead and begun screening blood with a surrogate test.

Strategically, federal decisions were essential to the Red Cross's uniform national defense strategy. National standards, rather than state or local ones, were more likely to be employed by federal courts. Since there were fewer federal courts, a favorable verdict would have a precedent-setting domino effect. The Kozup suit had already helped the Red Cross build a successful defense portfolio in those areas. To that end, it attempted to have state cases moved to federal court.

The debate over which court—federal or state—had jurisdiction over the Red Cross had resulted in more than forty different district court rulings. In mid-1992, for the first time the Supreme Court had the opportunity to resolve the issue. The case concerned a New Hampshire woman identified in the suit as SG, who had had a hysterectomy in Concord Hospital in 1984. During that operation she had been transfused with blood from Red Cross's Vermont–New Hampshire region. *SG v. the American Red Cross,* which also named the by-then deceased surgeon and a surgical products manufacturer, had been brought in New Hampshire State Court.

The Red Cross argued that as an instrumentality of the United States, it had the right to be heard by a federal judge. SG's lawyer countered that federal court would require that each defendant be sued separately. That would enable the Red Cross to use the "empty chair defense": each jury would think the absent "other" defendant was to blame. The "other" in this case could conveniently be the deceased surgeon. The cost to bring such a suit on a defendant-by-defendant basis would be time consuming and expensive for the AIDS victim, who had limited time and money.

"Everyone thinks there's some hidden or sinister motive," said one of the attorneys for the Red Cross. "We're simply trying to get uniformity in the way these cases are decided. We don't want to be in one court in California and another in Alabama. This is one way of trying to manage a difficult docket."

To reinforce its position, the Red Cross enlisted the U.S. Justice Department, which had come to its aid during the Abbott Labs AIDS kit controversy. Justice submitted an amicus ("friend of the court") brief in support of the Red Cross's motion to remove the SG case to federal court. The government attorneys cited, as justification, the Red Cross's performance of "a wide variety of functions indispensable to the workings of our Armed Forces . . . and to assist the federal government in providing disaster assistance."

In June, the Supreme Court granted the Red Cross the right to remove transfusion-AIDS lawsuits to federal court. By year end, the organization would win favorable decisions—largely summary judgment (dismissal), based on its "standard of care" defense in virtually every transfusion-AIDS case brought before a federal judge. In a typical decision which had multiple state reverberations, an Eastern District judge in Pennsylvania prevented a hemophiliac from taking the Red Cross and Baxter Healthcare to trial. The judge determined that blood banks could not be subject to the same legal standards as product manufacturers. The Red Cross had "complied with the applicable standard of care" during the first few years of the AIDS epidemic, and thus could not be sued for negligence.

That ruling would be binding for the entire 3rd U.S. Circuit, which included Pennsylvania, New Jersey, Delaware, and the U.S. Virgin Islands.

The victim's attorney, Philip Rush of Rush & Seiken, called the decision "devastating" and "appalling. This kills every case. I'm sure the Red Cross is going to be popping champagne corks tonight."

Such blanket rulings prompted the Association of Trial Lawyers of America's AIDS Litigation Group (ATLA) to dub federal court a "doomsday machine" for transfusion-AIDS cases.

The SG decision was just one of the hurdles government lawyers in tandem with the Red Cross had created for transfusion-AIDS victims. Another was in the area of expert witnesses.

For years, victims' attorneys had been unsuccessfully petitioning courts to allow testimony from key government officials. Specifically, plaintiffs sought out CDC experts like Don Francis who had alerted blood bankers about AIDS in early January 1983 and advised preventive measures. But by 1989, government lawyers from the U.S. Department of Health and Human Services had resisted at least fifty such requests or subpoenas from plaintiff lawyers.

Health and Human Services claimed that CDC employees would be unable to fulfill their disease-fighting mission were they to spend their time in court. In addition, allowing CDC testimony would ostensibly violate the government's policy of strict neutrality in private litigation.

The Red Cross, however, appeared to be exempt from such restrictions. In a 1987 transfusion-AIDS case, it was allowed to call as an expert witness a CDC official who had *not* been present at the fateful January 4, 1983 meeting. That official downplayed the blood industry's knowledge of AIDS transmissibility through blood. The Red Cross won on summary judgment and the case was dismissed without trial.

In May 1992, the Red Cross was not held to government policy when it faced its first trial in a transfusion-AIDS case. The suit was brought in Cleveland, Ohio, by a seventy-one-year-old woman who had been transfused with infected blood during surgery in 1983. Red Cross's Arnold & Porter counsel Peter Bleakley argued that the medical community had been divided and confused in 1983 as to what action to take about AIDS. Bleakley told the jury that the Red Cross did not believe the surrogate blood test was workable. The Red Cross also did not believe donors would be honest in answering questions about their sex lives. In a classic "empty chair" defense, the Red Cross blamed the doctor, who had settled out of court, for not informing the patient of transfusion risks.

Bleakley's argument was supported by the expert testimony of Dr. Harvey Klein, chief of transfusion services at the National Institutes of Health. Like CDC, NIH is a division of the Department of Health and Human Services. Presumably, NIH would be bound by the same rules as CDC. Not so—at least, not for the Red Cross. Klein was allowed to testify in the Red Cross's defense: he offered his expert opinion that lab tests for AIDS were of unknown value in 1983.

When questioned, jurors said that they felt the Red Cross might have done some things differently, but that it had not been negligent. They had given much weight to the NIH testimony.

By early 1992, Dr. Don Francis was no longer affiliated with CDC, and no longer subject to the dictates of government lawyers. He had left CDC's Atlanta headquarters in 1985 after his proposal to prevent AIDS had been "scoffed and trivialized" at a government meeting in Washington, D.C. By 1984, AIDS had been ranked in virulence with Class 4 viral agents, what Francis called "the big time mothers: Ebola, Lassa fever, hemorrhagic fevers. 'Hot zone' stuff." His Operation AIDS Control prevention plan would have cost the government $37 million. A small price, he thought, to save countless lives.

"Instead of being told to activate the plan," Francis later recalled, "we were told, 'Look pretty and do as little as possible.' That was not what I was trained for at CDC, to sit back and watch an epidemic burn."

Francis, his physician wife and two sons went west. He retained his affiliation with CDC as special consultant and instituted in California one of the nation's most advanced HIV prevention programs. By early 1992, the epidemiologist had built an impressive record in AIDS prevention as CDC's adviser to the Department of Health Services for the State of California, special CDC consultant on AIDS to the City and County of San Francisco, and CDC's regional AIDS consultant for the U.S. Public Health Service in San Francisco. He had also represented the World Health Organization on an infectious disease project in the Sudan.

Over the years Francis had kept abreast of litigation developments in transfusion AIDS. To him, it was bad enough that these people had suffered, let alone had to seek redress through the courts. Perhaps the fear of litigation, and its costs, would force blood bankers into future accountability. Certainly CDC had failed to compel the industry by recommendation. FDA had failed by regulation. And plain ethics seemed to have fallen somewhere along the wayside.

In early 1992, Francis retired from CDC to work on his longtime dream: developing an AIDS prevention vaccine. Initially he contracted with the biotech company Genetech, then went on to found a separate division within the company. At the end of February, he teamed with Jonas Salk, the polio vaccine pioneer. It was then that Francis received a packet in the mail from an attorney in North Carolina who was suing the Red Cross on behalf of a transfusion-AIDS victim.

It was only with cursory interest that Francis began reading the enclosed deposition of a high-level Red Cross official, a key decision maker during the early 1980s. Within minutes his attention was riveted. The official had testified under oath that CDC's data in 1983 had been insufficient to warrant blood bank action against AIDS, that the CDC had not known AIDS was infectious, that no one then had really known much at all about blood-borne AIDS. And on and on.

That's when it struck Francis: the industry had learned nothing over the years. It was still mired in the kind of institutional arrogance that had cost innocent people their lives. It was continuing to plead ignorance and to malign the "messenger," CDC, because it did not like the message. Because the truth would cost money and did not fit into their orderly pre-AIDS universe.

The lawlessness of it was insupportable.

"I came in with both barrels," Francis said of his agreeing to testify in the North Carolina case. "Then I ended up taking on the burden."

Several attorneys from Arnold & Porter deposed him. The one-day deposition lasted eleven hours in a hotel room in San Francisco on an unusually steamy day. Francis had spent most of his life working as a member of a team. He was used to pulling together to achieve a common goal, hashing out disagreements, refining extremities, keeping a positive, productive momentum going. He was not prepared for the kind of aggressive questions with which the Red Cross sought to undermine what he had accomplished, what he stood for, who he was. "I had never been attacked like that in public before. It was shocking."

After the sixth hour of repetitive questions, it dawned on Francis what the attorneys were attempting to do: "They were trying to exhaust me so I'd never want to do this again in my life. They wanted to get me out of these cases for good."

The lawsuit did not go to trial. But when a later case against a blood bank did go to trial in July 1992 while Francis was attending an AIDS conference in Amsterdam, he made sure his voice was heard: his testimony was videotaped, and he returned for in-court rebuttal.

For transfusion-AIDS victims, *Quintana v. United Blood Services* was a landmark. The basis of the Quintana tragedy was no different from most transfusion-AIDS cases: a surgery patient had received HIV contaminated blood in 1983. But its process of resolution and outcome were markedly different.

Susie Quintana, an Hispanic woman in Southwest Colorado, had been the victim of an accidental gunshot wound. In 1985, when she learned she was HIV positive, she decided to sue the Phoenix-based blood provider, United Blood Services (UBS), the second largest blood provider after the Red Cross. "This was a very soft-spoken fighter with a lot of guts and determination to fight this out," recalled Bruce Jones of his first meeting with Mrs. Quintana. The young attorney with Holland & Hart, one of the largest law firms in the Rocky Mountain region, knew little about AIDS and nothing about transfusion-associated AIDS. The Quintana case would launch him into a decade of battling blood banks, including the Red Cross.

Mrs. Quintana's claim was negligence: UBS had not properly screened blood donors in 1983 and it had not implemented surrogate testing. Her case was tried twice. In 1988, the first trial court judge excluded expert testimony that criticized prevailing practices among blood bankers. Among those critics were Drs. Marcus Conant, the San Francisco AIDS specialist, and Edgar Engleman, director of the Stanford Blood Bank. They were prepared to tell the jury that the industry's screening and testing procedures in 1983 had been substandard, that methods had indeed been available which would have identified the infected unit. But Conant and Engleman were limited in their testimony.

Furthermore, the judge instructed the jury that UBS could not be found negligent if it complied with the standard of care, defined as the customs and practices of the industry at the time of Quintana's transfusion. "Professional medical negligence" could be proved as a matter of law only if UBS had deviated from the accepted standard. UBS had not. As such, the jury had had no choice but to render a verdict for UBS.

Holland & Hart appealed the decision on the grounds that the judge erred in applying the professional medical standard to UBS. He had prevented the plaintiffs from presenting evidence that would have shown that the industry's customs and practices might not have been reasonable and prudent. And he had wrongly instructed the jury that if UBS had complied with those standards it could not be found negligent. Holland & Hart won their appeal in early 1992, and the case was retried in July.

On his return from Amsterdam, during rebuttal in court, Don Francis explained to the jurors what had transpired at the decisive January 4, 1983 meeting. CDC had presented data indicating the risk of blood-borne AIDS and the high-risk gay donors. CDC had told the blood industry that surrogate testing, specifically hepatitis anti-core, would screen out a high percent of high-risk donors and that gay men should not be giving blood.

Francis told the court, "It was very clear. "If there was any consensus between us, CDC and the blood bankers, it was that gay and bisexual men should be excluded from donating blood."

As for surrogate testing, "We knew for the better part of a decade that hepatitis B was a major epidemic in gay men. It was a very useful marker for homosexuality, or at least behavior in homosexual men that put them at risk for HIV infection. We presumed you'd prevent seventy, eighty percent of the AIDS infection by using hepatitis B markers."

Not 100 percent, but a solid step along the way, part of the process of what, to Francis, science was all about: "Just trying to get to the truth of the situation."

The blood bankers rejected CDC's advice, Francis told the jury. "We had a natural experiment going on. And as a result, Susie Quintana was infected, as are several thousand individuals in this country because of, I think, a decision that was made that was inappropriate."

On July 31, as Holland & Hart attorney Maureen Witt was delivering closing remarks, a message was handed the court: Susie Quintana had died of AIDS complications. During lunch, UBS and Quintana's attorneys met in the judge's chambers. UBS moved for a mistrial. The judge refused, but he ordered the jury sequestered: it was not to know about Mrs. Quintana's death because of possible prejudicial effects. This sequestering of a civil court jury was a first for Denver.

On August 1, Susie Quintana won her case. Whereas in 1984, the Red Cross had officially assessed the value of a human life lost from transfusion AIDS at $500,000, the jury awarded $8.5 million to Quintana for her pain and suffering and to her husband for his loss of consortium. Only then did the jury learn Mrs. Quintana had died the day before.

The Quintana case thrust Holland & Hart into the transfusion-AIDS spotlight. By the summer of 1992 the firm was handling about ten such cases, most of which had been brought against the Red Cross. For Bruce Jones and Maureen Witt and their associate, Steve Choquette, suing the Red Cross initially required a leap of faith. "You're dealing with a totally different persona," Jones explained. "The Red Cross is largely identified with Mom, apple pie, and the American way. UBS didn't have any of those bells and whistles. The public perception is that the Red Cross rides to the rescue when catastrophe hits, that they are only out to do good for the public." It would, Jones knew, be difficult to convey that "even though the Red Cross was not for profit, financial considerations were something that factored into their analysis."

In Choquette's view, "The Red Cross wanted to do everything in its ability to assure plaintiff counsels representing transfusion-associated AIDS were hampered in their ability to share information and coordinate their strategy because of protective orders sealing prior case documents."

Chris Tisi had contacted Holland & Hart upon learning of the Quintana victory. He and Choquette began a supportive information-sharing relationship to the extent the court order allowed.

The Red Cross was beginning to face the legal fallout from victims who had acquired AIDS after testing began. Like Robert Jones, who had received HIV-infected blood in Portland, Oregon during a 1989 transfusion; a Reston, Virginia man who had contracted AIDS following a 1986 stomach ulcer operation; and a New Jersey man who had received HIV-infected blood that same year during elective surgery. A case in Alabama offered some insight into Red Cross's potential defense strategy for transfusion AIDS contracted in the late 1980s.

The Alabama lawsuit was brought by a woman who had been admitted for treatment at the Southeast Alabama Medical Center in July, 1988 and received blood provided by the American Red Cross. In June, 1990, the Red Cross discovered the donor had tested positive for HIV. It did not notify the Medical Center of the donor's HIV status until December, 1990. In January, 1991, the woman was informed by her doctor of the donor's HIV status; she subsequently tested positive as well. In July, 1991 she filed the lawsuit. After two years of complex legal argument under existing state liability law and statutorily required standard of care, the Red Cross was successful in obtaining summary judgement dismissing the lawsuit. Although the court observed that the woman and her family had suffered a great tragedy, it concluded that the facts presented did not warrant relief under the law.

Meanwhile Roland Ray's class action suit had been dealt a blow in mid-1992. The District of Columbia Superior Court in Washington, D.C. determined that each victim—as many as 235—must bring separate suits. Roland decided to proceed on his own. The complaint was amended and refiled.

Mike Feldman and his "Red Cross SWAT Team" began shoring up their list of expert witnesses: Stanford's Edgar Engleman, San Francisco's Marcus Conant, and Dr. Don Francis, who told Mike Feldman that he would be delighted to take the stand on behalf of Roland Ray.

CHAPTER TWELVE

FOUR CHILDREN

The Red Cross should get down on its knees and beg forgiveness.

Dr. Don Francis

It seemed to Jewelle Michaels that Jim was taking pictures of every single minute of the girls' lives—pictures and videos of them in their pink tutus dancing to "Great Balls of Fire," playing "Amazing Grace" on the piano, jumping over foaming surf on Virginia Beach, watching TV, eating, resting, and sleeping. As Heather grew weaker, Jim's picture-taking took on an urgency. It both saddened and terrified Jewelle. Jim seemed to be trying to stop the clock, hold back time—keep the girls frozen in their moments of peace and happiness.

By year end 1991, Heather could no longer attend school. She had been hospitalized twice at the University of Virginia Medical Center for severe pneumonia. New lesions had since appeared. They were resistant to acyclovir and persisted for two-week stretches over the course of several months. Half blind, she developed severe herpes infections. Progressive neurological damage had begun.

On January 15, 1992 Jim met with George Murdock, superintendent of the elementary school. The girls were outstanding students, cheerful and well liked, and the tragic news came as a shock to Murdock. He immediately recognized the potential for anxiety and confusion in this insulated rural community.

Murdock spoke at length with Dr. Frank Saulsbury. The physician assured him that if the girls' condition had imperiled the school environment in any way, he would long ago have advised their withdrawal. Murdock told Saulsbury that the school board would be called on to address the unique situation. Jim decided that Hailey and Holly would remain at home until the issue was resolved.

The following day, Murdock sent out several hundred letters to parents, informing them that the school had "a case of HIV positive this year" and that the child was no longer attending school. Murdock wrote, "As you know, the medical profession states that HIV cannot be contracted through 'casual contact.' I want to make parents aware of the case so that they may receive first-hand information rather than deal with rumors." A public meeting was planned for January 21.

To prepare the staff, Murdock asked a local pediatrician to discuss the disease with the teachers and answer any questions. On the evening of the twenty-first, George Murdock told a packed room of about 300 parents, "The main thing we're trying to do is educate everybody as quickly as we can. We feel the fear of the unknown is far greater than the fear of the known."

A review committee was formed. Murdock did not know how long the process would last and suggested Jim consider enrolling his daughters at another nearby elementary school "to prevent any possibility of other students and parents becoming aware of her illness." Jim decided to wait out the review.

Meanwhile, Heather grew worse. She ran fevers, lost weight, and experienced night sweats. Varicella, a chronic form of chicken pox, recurred. Holly and Hailey gathered around their sister, who was spending more time in bed, and Jewelle saw how sad they were for Heather to be hurting.

"I'm sorry you don't feel good, Sissy," they told her. "Can I do anything for you? I'll be right here."

Heather had trouble speaking. Her voice often slurred, so she just smiled.

Jim told Murdock to focus on returning Holly to school since Hailey was experiencing medical problems and might be home a while. Saulsbury assured Murdock that Holly had no excessive bruising or bleeding and required no medication that had to be administered during the schoolday. "She has enjoyed good health," he wrote to Murdock. "My recommendations for Holly in terms of school are quite simple. She should be treated like every other student in the school. She poses absolutely no risk to other students or staff. Likewise, the other students and staff pose no threat to Holly."

It was not until March that Hailey was able to return to school. She had been treated with a new antiviral drug which resulted in complete resolution of her varicella. By then, Holly was happily ensconced in her second-grade class.

In May, Heather was hospitalized for AIDS-related problems. Her speech worsened. Saulsbury wrote to Murdock that the child was too sick to continue her homebound instruction.

Heather's body hurt even to the slightest touch. "You tired, doll baby?" Jewelle would ask. "Want Granny to hold you a little while?" Jewelle would sit on the couch and place the softest pillow on her lap. Her granddaughter would lie across it and rest.

Once, when Heather was half asleep, her eyes flew open and she looked up, far off, past her grandmother. It seemed to Jewelle that Heather was looking at something only she could see. Then Heather reached up with her right arm, and stretched it out as if she were trying to grab on to something.

It was an angel, Jewelle thought. Heather had seen an angel.

When Jim was not working double shifts, he was reading about AIDS. One article in particular stayed in his mind. It seemed that all HIV blood had hepatitis in it, he explained to his mother. Blood centers were supposed to be screening for hepatitis, so why did the girls get sick? Their medical bills were soaring. Basic expenses were about $150,000 a year for each girl, not counting increasing hospitalization for Heather.

"Somebody messed up somewhere," Jim said. Whoever they were, he wanted them to pay for what they'd done to his girls.

Jim called several local attorneys, asking whether he had a case. They had no idea what, if anything, he could do. Then, in late spring, a friend referred him to Tom Current. Current ran a small practice in Lynchburg. He told Jim that he would do some legal research and see if there was a case, and if so, against whom.

A number of transfusion-AIDS cases involving children had recently entered the court system. One was brought by a mother whose three hemophiliac sons had died of AIDS, all within a four-year period. The Tucson, Arizona suit charged nine Factor VIII manufacturers, the Red Cross, and several local hospitals with negligence. In Bucks County, Pennsylvania, the parents of a thirteen-year-old girl filed suit against the Red Cross and four implicated blood donors, identified only by their Red Cross–assigned numbers. The girl, "Mary Doe," had received blood transfusions at the ages of two, five, eight, and twelve. She learned she was HIV positive in 1991. The suit accused the Red Cross of inadequately preventing the spread of AIDS through its blood supply.

The mother of a hemophiliac boy filed suit in Illinois against two blood supply companies and, the Red Cross's St. Louis chapter for having failed to screen donors and properly test and process blood supplies. The boy, ten-year-old Keith Croffoot, made news in 1987 when he won a court battle to remain in school. He wanted, he said, "to teach people not to be afraid of AIDS."

A far more public figure had brought transfusion AIDS back into the news in the spring of 1992. Tennis player Arthur Ashe announced during a news conference that he had AIDS. He was "ninety-five percent sure" that his infection had been the result of a transfusion he had received in 1983, after heart bypass surgery.

Ashe's revelation prompted a flood of calls to the national AIDS hotline. The Red Cross assured the public that chances of contracting AIDS from blood were no more than one in 225,000. One longtime employee took to the airways, defending the Red Cross. Dr. Gerald Sandler still served as medical director of the Red Cross. He was also associated with Georgetown University Hospital. Sandler told National Public Radio, "A lot of people say, well, if you did something at ten in the morning, couldn't you have done it at nine and wouldn't that have been better? There was no test for the AIDS virus before there was a test for the AIDS virus. About five people in every hundred would have had to have been told at that time, 'The American Red Cross and the federal Food and Drug Administration and so forth find that your blood is so much at risk for the AIDS virus that we didn't transfuse it.' Now, that test would have caused an epidemic of fear and panic in the United States in the years 1983 and 1984, far greater than the AIDS virus itself."

Sandler was adamant that "There was not a unit of blood that was known to have tested positive for the AIDS and hepatitis B virus that we released by error and transfused to an individual person."

A few weeks after Sandler's interview, the Red Cross was forced to recall hundreds of improperly tested blood units and blood products in ten states—California, Florida, Illinois, Kentucky, Oklahoma, Ohio, New Jersey, Pennsylvania, South Carolina and West Virginia—and Switzerland, where product had been exported. Despite Elizabeth Dole's Transformation plan and Congressional inquiries, government inspections revealed that there were still serious questions of compliance with federal law by the Red Cross.

Transformation 1992 had been making its way through the blood regions, but its promises were short on delivery. There were still no new measures in place to ensure blood safety, no advanced technologies by which to track donors and recipients, no centralized computerization, no local biomedical boards or increased internal inspections by Red Cross personnel. Mrs. Dole's much-heralded employee education and training program had since translated into one- to two-day pep talks that over time substantially diminished in duration.

In fact, conditions and practices in 1992 at Red Cross facilities remained perilous. In Los Angeles, FDA discovered that 33 blood products had been manufactured from donations from individuals with a history of hepatitis. Donors testing reactive for HIV had not been deferred until years later. Look-Back of suspected post-transfusion AIDS had not been performed for many years in 97 cases. The FDA noted that "Prompt notification was needed to prevent secondary transmission of HIV." The Rochester, New York center was temporarily closed when 150 "errors" were found in the screening of blood. A recall of 171 components manufactured from that suspect blood had been initiated. In Nashville, at least 1,200 lab records on HIV and hepatitis tests, antibody screening, quarantine status, and blood typing were missing, lost, or otherwise unavailable for inspection. In Buffalo, where the Red Cross held AIDS prevention workshops as part of Worlds AIDS Day, 1,896 blood components had been manufactured from contaminated blood and released for use that year. In Farmington, Connecticut, 29 whole blood units were drawn from donors deferred because of a history of hepatitis, use of IV drugs, or HIV-reactive test results.

In the Greater Chesapeake and Potomac region, there were approximately 6,000 discrepant records, making donor/recipient traceback virtually impossible. Of 250 error and accident reports, 83 had not been submitted to Red Cross headquarters in a timely manner.

The Tri State region in Huntington, West Virginia, found itself in a particularly hot seat. The region had to recall 350 questionable blood units and products. FDA had also discovered 1,313 discrepant donor files. In addition, 47 donors who had tested reactive for HIV between 1985 and 1987 had not been properly deferred, among them a donor who had been implicated in a 1985 transfusion-AIDS case.

Tri State blood had been the source, years earlier, of Anthony Kirby's transfusion AIDS.

For the Kirby family, 1992 was a trying year. For Connie, it was a time of gathering her internal resources to cope with knowing her son, Anthony, was going to die. When she and her husband learned about Anthony's diagnosis, they had gathered together their closest friends and church pastor and told them. The support was overwhelming. They met with the principal of the elementary school and gave him permission to inform Anthony's teacher. When Connie and Darrell told Anthony's older brother, Mat, they all cried together.

Connie knew she was angry. But she also knew that she could not live in anger. It would be like a cancer eating her up inside. Darrell's rage, though, was unmitigated. It wasn't right, he told his wife. The surgeon had not even told them about Anthony's transfusion. Darrell wanted to sue the doctor. He contacted a local law firm, Caldwell, Cannon-Ryan & Riffee, and spoke with Joe Caldwell. Caldwell said he would explore whether the Kirbys had a case. A few weeks later, while Anthony was suffering a bout of lesions that had attacked his tongue and mouth, Caldwell called. He told Darrell, "This is bigger than we thought." It was far too much for his firm to handle. But he had come across attorneys in Colorado who had recently won a major transfusion-AIDS lawsuit. Caldwell had spoken with one of them, Steve Choquette. Choquette and his firm were interested in the Kirbys' case.

In December, Anthony was hospitalized for AIDS-related pneumonia, retinitis, and excruciating pain in his legs. His mother remained in the hospital with him for a period of two months. By then he was wearing what the Kirbys called his "happy meal," an IV unit implanted under his skin through which he could receive essential nutrients. He had all but stopped eating. A second IV unit, this one for morphine drops to help alleviate the pain, had also been implanted.

Anthony was very angry. He alternated between screaming and crying. Connie sensed he knew he was very ill and that his outbursts were rooted in fear and frustration. Dr. Saulsbury suggested she talk to him about his illness; that might alleviate the anxiety of the unknown. In preparation, Connie stayed up late one night in the room reserved for parents in the pediatric wing and prayed. Then she took a long shower, and in the shower she cried.

The next morning, she read Anthony his favorite Berenstain Bears book. She sat on the hospital bed, Anthony's head on her lap, gently stroking his head. Even listening tired him. She decided to bring up the subject of his illness. Softly, Connie began explaining that he was very sick. He might get a little better, but he would get sick again. Connie wiped the tears she could not stop, but some still fell on Anthony's blond hair. She asked him if he wanted to know the name of his sickness.

Anthony lay quietly for a while.

"No," he finally said.

After that, Anthony seemed calmer. He talked about going to Chuck E Cheese, a pizza place where kids could play video games for quarters. For the past few months, his school friends had been sending Anthony quarters, an incentive to get well. Anthony had, he told his mother, over $100 in quarters. Couldn't they go? One mild afternoon, Connie, Darrell, Anthony's brother, Mathew, and two off-duty nurses who had become attached to their young patient sneaked him out of the hospital. They picked up his two best friends and his favorite aunt Margaret and went to Chuck E Cheese.

Anthony was wearing his "happy meal" and his morphine drip, but that did not stop him from playing all the games. When he had exhausted his bounty of quarters, a man standing nearby handed Margaret what she thought was a dollar. Without a second glance, she gave it to Anthony. He shrieked in delight. It was a fifty-dollar bill.

When Margaret turned to thank the man, he was gone. Connie was not surprised. That was how people responded to Anthony. He was a very special child.

It was during that hospital stay that Steve Choquette, accompanied by a Holland & Hart partner, Harold "Sonny" Flowers, flew to Roanoke, West Virginia, to meet the Kirbys. Nine-year-old Anthony was their youngest transfusion AIDS client, and both men were deeply affected by what they saw. The boy was shockingly pale and frail, but he had an astonishing sweetness, a vigorous spirit. When the attorneys prepared to leave, Anthony hugged them both goodbye. Later, the hefty 6´5˝ Flowers told Choquette, "I almost lost it."

The Kirby lawsuit charged the Red Cross with failing to implement donor screening, failing to properly test donated blood with at least one surrogate test for the causative agent of AIDS, and failing to properly screen donors according to its own policies and standards. Other charges were related to the Red Cross's failure to revise donor history procedures and its failure to issue instructions and guidelines to its Tri State blood center concerning questions designed to recognize the early signs of AIDS. The suit also claimed that the Red Cross failed to properly educate physicians about AIDS transmission via blood and that it did not encourage physicians and hospitals to allow autologous or directed donations.

As a result of the Red Cross's negligence and its communications failures with Tri State and the local hospital, whose surgeon and anesthesiologist were also named in the suit, Anthony contracted AIDS, became seriously ill, and suffered extreme physical pain.

The surgeon was specifically charged with not complying with his contract with the Kirbys to "reuse Anthony's blood should a transfusion be needed."

Holland & Hart was inundated with motions from Red Cross's counsel, Arnold & Porter.

In an attempt to quash the Kirby suit, Arnold & Porter moved for summary judgment—dismissal for lack of merit citing the Red Cross's traditional defense: conformity with the blood industry's standard of care in 1983 and 1984. That meant no direct questioning of donors and no surrogate blood tests. But the Red Cross's standard-of-care defense did not persuade the judge in the Kirby case that a jury trial was precluded. The court ruled that prevailing industry practice did not exempt the Red Cross from facing trial.

With the path cleared for victim claims, the Red Cross requested sovereign immunity. While it could be subject to trial, the Red Cross argued that as an "instrumentality" of the government, it was not required to face a jury trial or pay punitive damages. Again, the Kirby judge decided otherwise: the Red Cross would be subject to jury trial and to punitive damages if the claimants prevailed.

Twice thwarted, the Red Cross requested removal of the case to the federal courts, a right it won.

The Red Cross proceeded to file objections to producing the documents requested by Choquette, and it moved to restrict expert testimony on behalf of the victims. Choquette recalled, "They never answered a single request for information without preceding the answer with voluminous legal objections. Getting complete documents was a dogfight." Choquette was forced to filing motions to compel the Red Cross to respond. "They were incredibly careful," Choquette said. "They'd white out documents, correspondence, Look-Back files, anything that gave the slightest lead to the donors' identity."

The battle to compel the Red Cross to provide information on donors' identities implicated in transfusion-AIDS cases had long been an arduous one for plaintiffs' attorneys. Faced with often insurmountable legal objections that required time and money, victims had resorted, in some cases, to desperate measures. In a Michigan transfusion-AIDS case, for instance, the Red Cross had won a protective order barring the victim's access to information identifying the donor. But the donor's social security number had inadvertently been left on the Red Cross registration card. The plaintiff's attorney hired a private investigator, who discovered the donor's name and the fact that he was an active homosexual. The court was not pleased at this violation of the protective order. It not only imposed sanctions against the victim, Cheryl Coleman, it dismissed her case against the Red Cross. Coleman was also barred from suing the donor. But an appeals court overturned the latter ruling, and she was permitted to pursue legal action against the donor, who had allegedly displayed overt negligence in donating blood.

The Red Cross knew how damaging identifying an implicated donor could be. In the case of Bob Jones, the Montana carpenter who had received HIV-tainted blood in 1989 at the Portland, Oregon center, the Red Cross had argued that the blood had tested negative. It also claimed that Portland had properly screened the donor. Despite the Red Cross's effort to prevent donor discovery, Jones's attorney located the donor. The man did not fit Portland's description. He was willing to testify that had he been directly questioned about his lifestyle, he would not have given blood. On the second day of the trial, before the donor took the stand, the Red Cross suddenly settled. It did not admit negligence, but it had the internal documents placed under protective order, effectively sealed from the view of other plaintiff attorneys.

In the Kirby case the judge compelled the Red Cross to disclose the donor's identification.

The Red Cross also refused to respond to Ashcraft & Gerel's request concerning donor identity in the triplets case, which the firm had taken on in late 1992. It had, it claimed, retained a sample of the donor's blood, which was by then eleven years old. There was a question as to the accuracy of any test performed on that blood, and Feldman did not pursue further motions to identify the donor.

The Red Cross sought and won protective orders prior to trial in both the Kirby and Michaels' cases. "They did not want the public to see documents that indicate the depth and breadth of their knowledge of AIDS and what needed to be done early in the epidemic," Steve Choquette said.

On a cold January afternoon in 1993, the phone rang in Jewelle Michaels' home. It was Billy Ray Cyrus, the country singer. Cyrus had heard about the triplets and wanted to say hello.

"Can you put her on the phone, ma'am?" Cyrus asked Jewelle.

Jewelle explained to him that Heather could no longer speak. "But she can listen to you and she can communicate with you with her beeper. It has a kind of bell sound. You could ask her questions and she could beep 'yes' or 'no.' "

Jewelle took the phone to Heather's bed. Cyrus talked with her for a long time and Heather, her face pocked with lesions, was aglow. From time to time, she beeped back.

A few days later, Heather Michaels died of AIDS in her bed at home. Her father and grandmother were beside her. She was eight and a half years old.

CHAPTER THIRTEEN

DANGEROUS OPPORTUNITIES
1993

The American Red Cross has embodied much of what is best about Americans: their willingness to help their neighbors, to take responsibility for their communities, and to respond to the call of service.

President Bill Clinton

Following the 1991 congressional hearings, John Dingell was convinced that the Red Cross was taking FDA's voluntary agreement seriously. Elizabeth Dole's Transformation was admittedly ambitious, but in the face of potential federal shutdown of the nation's largest blood collector, drastic measures were called for.

During the prior two years, there had been a good deal of internal scrambling at the Red Cross: hirings and firings, a string of high-priced consultants, and changes in approaches, philosophies, deadlines, and costs. Tens of millions had already been spent designing a computer system that was not fully operational. Quality assurance had not materialized. Meanwhile, the Red Cross was falling further and further behind in implementing federal regulations.

Transformation was clearly not panning out quite the way Mrs. Dole had promised.

By 1993, Transformation had, in fact, become a matter of power: political power and the power of image.

Early on, Dr. William Swallow, vice president of the northeastern Pennsylvania board of directors, had had an intuitive sense that Transformation was about power, not about the needs of the Red Cross or the communities it served. In 1991, he had attended the annual meeting at which Elizabeth Dole announced Transformation. He wanted to be optimistic but had his doubts about Transformation. He questioned its viability and its motives.

When Bill Swallow moved to the small town of Milton, Pennsylvania in 1981 to join the staff of Geisinger Medical Center, he was asked to serve as medical director at the local Red Cross chapter. He'd always had a soft spot for the Red Cross. He respected their public service and was himself a six-gallon donor. In 1985, Swallow became chapter chairman, then filled an unexpired term on the board of the Regional Blood Center at Wilkes-Barre. He remained as its vice president.

Swallow had been peripherally aware of problems in other blood centers, particularly in Portland, Oregon. Wilkes-Barre, however, had one of the finest reputations nationally. Its hospital clients were pleased, the community was supportive, and staff and volunteers worked harmoniously.

But it was Transformation's business schematic which especially bothered Swallow. Mrs. Dole had explained that in order to pay for the program, headquarters would have to borrow about $100 million from the employee pension fund. The pension fund was fat; by then employees did not have to pay into it to keep it going. Still, dipping into employee money struck Swallow as an odd way of doing business, particularly when Mrs. Dole assured staff that they were not going to bankroll Transformation.

"My feeling," he later recalled, "was that they were developing a business strategy to centralize as much of the power at headquarters and disempower the regions and the volunteer board. That way they could gain a business advantage, could begin to impact areas where the Red Cross was not the buyer's choice, and gain more sharehold nationally."

For some reason, the Chinese term for "crisis" came to Swallow's mind: it was "dangerous opportunity."

By the time Transformation arrived at Wilkes-Barre, it lasted only a few hours. Tony Polk, former head of Blood Services for the Armed Forces had been hired to deliver Mrs. Dole's message of change. The retired Army colonel spoke to Wilkes-Barre's staff about the "need for Transformation." To Swallow, that implied better training and quality assurances. Even Wilkes-Barre could profit from improvements.

Polk's talk was long on rationales for change, short on substance. Then Polk left.

Swallow subsequently learned that employees would, after all, be footing at least some of the bill for Transformation: they would have to start paying into the pension fund.

To Dr. Swallow, Mrs. Dole's Transformation was all "smoke and mirrors."

Like Swallow, Dr. David Jenkins, director of the Louisville, Kentucky blood center, was facing cost problems. Headquarters had assumed the right to make key business decisions in his region. As a result, the cost of doing business was steadily increasing. His center had also been required by headquarters to export its blood to other areas, where higher prices could be had. Local employee and volunteer morale was dipping.

Still, when Mrs. Dole visited Louisville, Dr. Jenkins was impressed. "She's a spellbinder as a speaker. At certain points tears came to her eyes. She made many promises." But like Dr. Swallow, Jenkins did not see them materialize. He began talking to other blood region directors about Transformation. Were they as disappointed? What was their assessment of Mrs. Dole? One comment in particular stayed in his mind. "That speech she gave when she had tears in her eyes—well, I heard she cries at that same point every time."

By fiscal 1992, the Red Cross was running a deficit of $5 million. In its annual report, it cited the reason for this deficit as "the large investment being made in the blood program in order to transform operations and procedures." That increased spending was ostensibly channeled into better "testing and quality control functions, training and education, facility maintenance and improved technical equipment." In fact, a parade of expensive consultants helped boost Biomedical services' spending an additional $20 million.

But for all the increased expense, few safety or operational improvements had actually taken place. Mrs. Dole's two-year deadline to centralize computerization had been moved up yet another year, to 1995; actual deployment was anticipated for 1997. Since February, IBM consultants had been steering Joint Application Development (JAD) groups through the process of identifying Red Cross's business requirements. Andersen Consulting was still sketching out computer options and another team from KPMG Peat Marwick, a computer management firm, was overseeing initial planning.

"It felt," said a former board member in the Northeast region, "like the consultants were running the Red Cross."

Among the many high-priced advisers was Michael Goldfarb, Mrs. Dole's former DOT colleague. Goldfarb's specialty was federal aviation issues. Mrs. Dole viewed him as her business consultant, someone on whom she depended for financial and management issues and judgment about people.

Goldfarb had been called in to assist the Red Cross's new senior vice president for Blood Services, Fred Kyle, in implementing Transformation. Mrs. Dole's hiring of the highly respected pharmaceutical executive had been considered a coup. Kyle was senior U.S. executive with SmithKline Beecham, PLC, the large British-based pharmaceutical company. He had managed 21,000 employees who generated $4 billion in pharmaceutical sales. A cultured, well-spoken man with a reputation for integrity, Kyle took a substantial pay cut to join Mrs. Dole's Red Cross. He told the *New York Times* the opportunity was "a chance to use the skills I've been using in the private sector and a chance to pay back some of the good luck I've had."

Insiders predicted Kyle would encounter the kind of resistance which had prompted his predecessor Jeffrey McCullough to leave. The question became: How long will Fred Kyle last aboard a ship whose captain is utterly dependent on a clique of progressively more powerful special mates?

Publicly, Mrs. Dole remained upbeat about her role at the Red Cross. In magazine and newspaper interviews she described her job as a logical extension of her work on Capitol Hill, but with a human touch.

"The part I love," she told to *Good Housekeeping* magazine, "is that you deal with dire human needs on a fulltime basis."

Meanwhile, she was building a power base which would mitigate increasing political pressures. In May, Norman Augustine, chief executive of Martin Marietta, the multibillion-dollar defense contractor, was named chairman of the Board of Governors of Red Cross. A longtime Washington insider and Liddy Dole fan, Augustine had held varied influential positions along the Beltway. He had been Undersecretary of the Army in the Ford administration, had chaired the Defense Science Board, which was dubbed the "ground zero" of the military-industrial complex, and had served under President Bush as chairman of the special White House committee on the future of the U.S. space program. Augustine had also chaired the U.S. Savings Bond Campaign to help raise money for a cash-strapped U.S. Treasury.

As the *Washington Post* characterized Augustine's influence, "In Washington power circles, there are two kinds of people. There are those who lobby. And there are the people who don't have to. Norman Augustine is one of those who doesn't have to."

Mrs. Dole's connection with Martin Marietta and Norm Augustine dated back to her early years at the Department of Transportation when Augustine was president of Marietta's aerospace division. That division became the first to benefit from a $10 billion National Airspace System Plan which Mrs. Dole announced in February 1984. Marietta's $684 million government contract would, she said, "help the FAA accomplish the entire plan on target."

Martin Marietta enjoyed further Liddy Dole patronage when, that year, Reagan created the Office of Commercial Space Transportation (OCST). Mrs. Dole wrested control of that office from the Commerce Department and placed it under DOT, naming her confidante, Jenna Dorn, as OCST's head. Martin Marietta won one of the first lucrative OCST contracts to convert Air Force Titan 2 ballistic missiles into expendable rocket launchers to send satellites into orbit. In 1986, the company would again profit from deregulation of the private space sector, an initiative Mrs. Dole hailed as "eliminating the government monopoly in space transportation."

The following year, her last at DOT, Mrs. Dole held a press conference with top Martin Marietta officials to announce a $220 million contract between Marietta and the International Telecommunications Satellite Organization (INTELSAT) to launch jointly two commercial satellites. "The Department of Transportation is proud to be able to assist commercial firms in making the economic frontier of space more accessible to development," Mrs. Dole said of the new alliance. She then appointed the president of Marietta's commercial rocket launch program head of DOT's Commercial Space Transportation Advisory Panel. A week later, Marietta became the first company to sign an agreement with the Air Force to use Defense Department facilities for commercial launches.

Mrs. Dole also lobbied for legislation limiting insurance liability for private firms like Marietta that were entering the commercial space market. When she left DOT to join her husband's 1988 presidential campaign, Jenna Dorn was hired by Martin Marietta as director of strategic planning.

Coincidentally, two of Bob Dole's top senatorial advisers were lobbyists for Lockheed-Martin, the product of Martin Marietta's merger with Lockheed.

Augustine's slot at the Red Cross was strictly voluntary. Money was not an issue: he earned over $4.2 million in 1992 from Martin Marietta, which claimed revenues of $6.1 billion. In 1993, Marietta nearly doubled its revenues by acquiring General Electric's aerospace business for $3.05 billion.

Mrs. Dole welcomed Augustine as "the visionary we need and can trust to spearhead our efforts as we take bold steps toward the next century." Among those steps was implementation of "our Blood Services Transformation, a far-reaching public safety program affecting half the nation's blood supply."

Augustine would donate directly to Bob Dole's 1996 presidency bid. So would members of Mrs. Dole's Board of Governors also support, either directly or indirectly, Bob Dole's political aspirations. In fact, Mrs. Dole had been buttressing her Board and "Members at Large" category with monied individuals, many of whose corporate or personal finance interests would be served by Bob Dole and the Republican Party.

Historically, the president of the Red Cross was accountable to the Board of Governors in policymaking matters. Mrs. Dole explained the difference between government and philanthropy: "Instead of carrying forward the policies of the President . . . an executive in the nonprofit sector has to work to inform the board, to advise, to recommend, and then carry forward the policies of the board." But by courting individuals and companies which, to varying degrees, relied on her husband's legislative policies, Elizabeth Dole was assured of unquestioned authority.

Among Mrs. Dole's newly acquired board members were officers with such companies as: Bell South, Martin Marietta, Nationwide Insurance, Sumitomo Sitx (real estate), and VISA. All would give to Bob Dole's presidential bid in 1996. Even Red Cross contractor Abbott Labs, which supplied its AIDS tests, would, through one of its executives, contribute to Dole for President.

Some Red Cross Board members, including United Technologies, have shown their support to Bob Dole through other less direct channels, including contributions to Bob Dole's Campaign America, a leadership PAC. PAC (political action committee) funds cannot be used directly for a candidate's campaigns. Rather, PACs are springboards from which a candidate can launch into higher office. "PAC money culls favors, buys 'chits,' " explained Shiela Krumhold, project director for the Center for Responsive Politics. "PACs are a form of 'slush fund,' another pocket of a politician's coat. The formation of a PAC often signals a politician is setting the stage for a jump to higher office, from Senate to President, for instance."

United Technologies provided financial support through their executives to Republican Party causes. So did Bell South, Nationwide, Martin Marietta, VISA, MAPCO Coal, Abbott Labs and Baxter Healthcare (which sold Red Cross plasma). Martin Marietta would contribute $118,750 to the National Republican Congressional and Senate Committees and $20,000 to the (Republican) President's dinner in 1994.

Mrs. Dole reeled in other heavyweight Bob Dole supporters: Atlantic Richfield Corporation and hometown Kansas Gas & Electric. She also brought into the "Members at Large" category her old friend Inez Andreas whose husband, Duane Andreas, head of Archer Daniels Midland, had first donated to the Red Cross when Mrs. Dole was named president. His second $500,000 accompanied his wife's appointment.

American Financial Corporation and a foundation tied to the insurance conglomerate American International Group, which supported the Red Cross's Gulf War Fund and backed Senator Dole's Foundation for the Disabled, also became big-money players for the Red Cross.

"They're stacking the deck," Dr. William Swallow observed. "You see all types of financial management decision making, which implies somebody's in trouble financially. It has to be in Red Cross's interest because certainly the money was needed. Is there a secondary gain, a secondary interest? I think there's a political interest there. There has to be. You can't close your eyes to that. These are mighty important, powerful people."

One former regional board chairman observed, "The board was there as a rubber stamp. They were chosen for their compliancy. They appeared to answer to her, rather than vice versa."

The way Louisville's Dr. David Jenkins saw it, "No one wants to alienate her [Mrs. Dole] if they have a contract with government, whether Bob Dole is Senate majority leader or President. I mean, the chairman of the Red Cross is the head of Martin Marietta, the biggest defense contractor." It seemed to him that Mrs. Dole's political ambitions had begun to dominate an organization whose founding principle was one of political neutrality. "They started functioning on a political paradigm, rather than a business paradigm. Like any political paradigm, image is everything. Results can

be presented in a variety of creative ways to make it look okay."
Meanwhile, he said, "The Red Cross was being run into the ground
by poor management and the American public was being poorly
served."

Mrs. Dole's clout would, however, serve her well. It would help her
escape, typically unscathed, when FDA lowered the boom in May
1993.

Negotiations had been proceeding in the Roland Ray case between Ashcraft & Gerel and Arnold & Porter, until an unexpected
turn of events encouraged the Red Cross to risk trial.

Compelled by court order to disclose the identity of Roland Ray's
donor, Arnold & Porter made that information available to Chris Tisi
and Mike Feldman through an intermediary or special master who
maintained the donor's anonymity in mid-1992. His anonymous deposition was planned for early December. Initially, Tisi and Feldman
felt fortunate that in this case the donor was still alive. Since he had
been HIV positive, he had likely been a high-risk candidate for AIDS.
They assumed that, had the Red Cross employed surrogate testing,
there would have been an 80 to 90 percent chance that Roland's
donor would have tested core positive. But Red Cross had not been
surrogate testing blood at that time. And it had not been directly
questioning donors about their high-risk lifestyles.

Mike Feldman and his team were confident they had a strong case
for negligence on both counts: failure of the Red Cross to use a surrogate test and its failure to take appropriate steps to screen high-
risk donors.

The deposition of Roland Ray's donor took place on December
1 and 3, in the presence of Mike Feldman, Chris Tisi, Peter Vangsnes,
and a young Ashcraft & Gerel associate, Sidney Schupak. Arnold &
Porter attorneys Bruce Chadwick, Fern O'Brian, and Terri Lavi represented the Red Cross. The donor was identified as "Mr. Donor."
The session was audiotaped for replay during trial.

"Mr. Donor" fit the typical profile of a Red Cross blood donor: he
was married, had children, and was a good citizen who felt a civic
responsibility to give blood. He had donated at least twenty-five
times during blood drives at his place of employment. In 1984, he
did not believe that he was at high risk for AIDS. He also did not
know that AIDS was sexually transmissible and fatal.

Feldman questioned Roland's donor about the Red Cross intake process at the time of his donation. How detailed had it been? How private? The donor explained that the routine questioning had taken place in a large, unpartitioned room, with no privacy. This, Feldman knew, was in violation of the Red Cross's own guidelines for conducting medical history interviews.

If he had been questioned about his sexual orientation in a confidential setting, what would he have answered? Feldman asked Mr. Donor.

"That I was bisexual," the donor said without hesitation.

He had done as much in 1985. That spring, when he again donated at work, the AIDS test was in use. He subsequently received a call from the medical director of the D.C. region, Fred Darr, who informed him of his test results. The donor recalled, "I was shocked." Darr asked if he would participate in a National Institutes of Health Study of HIV-positive men. He had agreed. When asked if he were a member of a high-risk group, he had responded that he was bisexual.

"If you had been told in 1984 that homosexual or bisexual men should not give blood, what would he have done?" Feldman asked.

"Not give it," the donor said. "I don't think I would have ever given blood. When I learned about it, [that] it was life threatening, and I was like—there's no way I wanted nobody to go through that."

Yes, he did recall a Red Cross pamphlet about donating blood. No, he had not read it. Like sixteen percent of Washington, D.C.'s population, Roland Ray's donor was functionally illiterate.

"Mr. Donor" figured that the Red Cross would tell him anything important he needed to know. He had thought, in 1984 , that his blood would be tested and was not told otherwise.

Roland's attorneys left the deposition feeling optimistic. A bisexual man who had not read the Red Cross pamphlet, the only screening barrier between HIV-infected donors and blood recipients, would, under confidential direct questioning, have disclosed his sexual lifestyle. Had he been directly informed of the high-risk categories, he would not have given blood.

Tisi and Feldman awaited the NIH records, which would also include surrogate blood test results.

Six weeks before trial, the NIH records arrived. Roland Ray's donor did not test positive on the surrogate blood test. "Mr. Donor" was among the ten or twenty percent of HIV-infected high-risk individuals who, for a variety of reasons, would have slipped through the blood screening. With that stunning news, Red Cross's failure to use the surrogate test, the centerpiece of most transfusion-AIDS cases, had suddenly become a moot point.

"It was," Tisi said, "very bad luck for Roland Ray."

Tisi, Feldman, and Vangsnes now knew that the jury would be hearing only half of the Roland Ray story. Their case would have to rest solely on Red Cross's failure to screen the donor adequately, a far more abstract charge to prove in court.

The news was an unexpected windfall for the Red Cross. "They did a 360-degree turn-around," Tisi recalled. "They knew that the surrogate test held real statistical weight that would be difficult to argue against. But proving a donor would have answered truthfully, that was a less tangible concept to convey to a jury. There was the human variable, which we would not have encountered with a blood test result."

Red Cross was indeed eager to go to trial, and Ashcraft & Gerel had to shift gears quickly. They would have to restructure Roland Ray's case at virtually the eleventh hour.

On May 3, 1993, the Superior Court of the District of Columbia called into session *Roland and Janet Ray v. the American National Red Cross.* Judge Richard Salzman presided. In one sense, Tisi, Feldman, and Vangsnes were pleased that Salzman was back on the bench. The judge had, in 1989, rendered the favorable Wilson decision, rejecting the Red Cross's standard of care argument and clearing the way for a trial. On the other hand, there was nothing to prevent Salzman from revisiting the issues and changing his mind.

Salzman summarized for the jury the Roland Ray case. Then began the process of voir dire: jury selection among sixty-six candidates. The nearly full-day process was indicative of AIDS's profound impact on society and the pervasive influence of the Red Cross. Many jurors were dismissed because they could not be impartial: they had either worked or volunteered for, donated blood to, or received some form of assistance from the Red Cross. Others were excused when they revealed that close friends or family had died of AIDS. In one case, a family member had died of transfusion AIDS. Another juror who had received blood transfusions in 1986 and 1989 explained: "I live in terror of AIDS"; she too was dismissed.

Still other jurors believed that the Red Cross should not be subject to such a lawsuit and that its stellar reputation would preclude their determining culpability. Others had had negative experiences with the organization during World War II.

It was late in the day by the time the jurors were finally selected and opening arguments began. For Chris Tisi, opening remarks provided an opportunity to tell his client's story and to troubleshoot. In this case, the first against the Red Cross which Ashcraft & Gerel would actually try, there was quite a bit of troubleshooting to do. Tisi had anticipated the Red Cross's arguments and intended to address them straight on.

Tisi briefed the jury on the chronology of the Red Cross's awareness of AIDS, beginning in 1982, when the CDC told blood bankers that AIDS was, most likely, blood borne. He recapped for them the January 4, 1983 meeting in which the Red Cross was told to screen out high-risk candidates for AIDS, namely, gay men. He talked about the government's recommendations that Red Cross adopt more stringent means to screen blood, including questioning donors in a confidential setting. All his claims would be supported by internal documents, he said. Those communications indicated that the Red Cross knew AIDS was transmissible by blood well over a year and a half before Roland Ray's transfusion. Yet the Red Cross had refused to act appropriately.

Anticipating the potential psychic resistance to impugning the Red Cross, Chris Tisi told the jury, "Now, I have to tell you up front that we have taken on a very large burden in this case. We are aware that the American Red Cross does some very good things. But like any person or organization, good or bad, organizations and people can make mistakes. And if you make mistakes, ladies and gentleman, the good person is just as responsible for the consequences as the person who is not so good."

On behalf of the Red Cross, Arnold & Porter counsel Peter Bleakley next addressed the jury. "From the very first time that people began to suspect that the AIDS disease could be transmitted by blood transfusion, the Red Cross began worrying about it," he told them. "Together with regulatory agencies, it began to try to develop ways to prevent people from contracting AIDS through blood transfusions." Ray's situation was admittedly tragic, but Bleakley explained, the first transfusion-associated AIDS case was reported in December 1982, "and there weren't a lot of people who weren't entirely sure even in that case if it had actually been caused by blood transfusion." The debate "continued into 1983 about whether in fact this was a blood-borne disease." By July 1984, "there were only about six transfusion-AIDS patients. There were none in the Washington metropolitan area. There was no test; no test became available for

AIDS until March of 1985, several months after this transfusion."

Bleakley told the jury that in 1983 and 1984, the Red Cross, the Council of Community Blood Centers, and the American Association of Blood Banks "considered whether or not . . . they should confront donors in some way about their sexual habits. And all decided against it. They decided against it because they thought it wouldn't work." Bleakley referred to threats by the gay community, and risks of blood shortages. "Red Cross and its peers decided not to do direct questioning in 1984 not because they didn't feel like it, but because they had nothing in mind but the health and welfare of the American people. The Red Cross agonized about the safety of the blood supply." Based on what they would hear, Bleakley told the jury, "you will conclude that the Red Cross acted responsibly, not negligently, and that its actions did not cause Mr. Ray to contract AIDS."

CHAPTER FOURTEEN

REASONABLE AND PRUDENT

May 1993

*Red Cross took advantage of its position and its power not
to fix what was broken. It's unconscionable to take a
favored position and hide behind it. I think that's evil.*

Leslie Vogt, President
Virginia Blood Services

As with most transfusion-AIDS cases, Roland Ray's hinged on a cir-
cular argument: the definition of "standard of care." Opposing counsels differed as to exactly what "standard of care" meant. The Red
Cross took the position that it had simply adhered to professional
customs and practices—that is, the prevailing practices of the industry. It did not fall below that standard and thus could not be
found negligent. On the other hand, Ashcraft & Gerel intended to
argue that the Red Cross *was* the industry. As the largest, most influential blood collector in the United States, the Red Cross was
looked to for leadership in setting the industry's prevailing practices.
The standard of care Red Cross set had been substandard. The industry's prevailing practices fell below what was reasonable and prudent. Since it had deviated from a reasonable standard of care,
Ashcraft & Gerel argued, the Red Cross could be found negligent.

Mike Feldman took over questioning from Chris Tisi.

The first witness was Dr. Don Francis. It would be the first transfusion AIDS trial against the Red Cross at which he would testify.
After establishing Francis's expertise in blood-borne diseases and
epidemics, Feldman moved to admit him as an expert witness. The
Red Cross counsel Peter Bleakley then questioned Francis. He
pointed out that Francis was not certified in blood banking, he was

not a member of any of the blood banking organizations, and had not worked at a blood bank. Francis had also not drafted donor screening procedures for any blood banks. Bleakley objected to Francis's designation as an expert. He would admit Francis as an expert in public health, epidemiology, or etiology for the transmission of AIDS, but not in the prevention of AIDS.

Feldman countered that AIDS was a public health issue that required the kind of expertise that blood bankers did not have. He told the judge, "There may be few people in the world that have as much knowledge about [AIDS] as Dr. Francis does." Francis had already explained in testimony the similarity between hepatitis and AIDS in mode of transmission, and that he had developed interview procedures for gay men to determine high-risk behavior. "The truth of the matter is, Your Honor, we are dealing with an AIDS epidemic and infectious disease epidemic. The expertise is how to deal with that epidemic."

Judge Salzman decided to permit Francis's testimony. "The jury needs [Francis's] assistance in these areas," he said. The term "expert," however, could not be used.

Feldman began building his case: what Red Cross, in fact, knew, versus its inaction based on that knowledge. He produced a photo he had had enlarged of the CDC meeting, and he placed it on an easel. Francis identified the individuals: Drs. Bruce Evatt, Jeff Koplan, and other CDC experts who were presenting information to the attending blood bankers. The subject was AIDS, high-risk donors, and the gay community. Francis explained, "CDC wanted to discuss potential ways that the unknown virus or unknown agent of AIDS could be prevented from being transmitted through the use of blood and plasma." CDC had conveyed the urgent need for blood bankers to address this crisis and it had prescribed means by which they could prevent the blood-borne transmission of AIDS, "relatively straightforward, logical ways of asking donors, specifically, male donors, if they'd had sex with other men." The transfusion cases were, Francis said, "absolutely critical because there was one exposure and then the onset of the disease. The concern was that the epidemic was far greater in reality than was apparent. If you can picture an iceberg, and we were looking just at the peak of this iceberg sitting at the top of the water," he said. The tip of that iceberg was "true AIDS." Below the surface were an unknown number of individuals incubating the disease.

Feldman then showed him Francis's letter. "It's an American Red

Cross memorandum from Dr. Cumming to Mr. deBeaufort, dated February 5, 1983."

Cumming was Red Cross's statistician, Arnie deBeaufort, the administrator of its AIDS Working Group. Cumming was responding to a memo which Blood Services director Fred Katz had sent to about sixteen of his officers about the potential of AIDS transmissibility through blood and gay donors. Feldman referred his witness to page four of the Cumming memo. After several objections by Peter Bleakley, Feldman was allowed to ask, "Is there anything in there regarding the subject of the incubation period [of AIDS]?"

"Yes," Francis replied. "It was clear that they understood what we were transmitting at the January meeting, that this was a long incubation period, estimated to be up to seven years at that time."

In the absence of a test, what would be the best means of screening potential donors to reduce the risk of AIDS?

"Basically, eliminate those donors that had behaviors that would put them at risk of getting infected." In addition to those infected with AIDS, Francis said, "that boiled down to gay and bisexual men."

Following the January 1983 meeting, did there exist, Feldman asked, a standard of care by which reasonable, prudent blood bankers would have, should have, responded to the screening of donors for AIDS?

"The meeting clearly set the standard of care. "Clearly there was an issue that AIDS was transmissible by blood and blood products and that the way to avoid that would be to have those at risk of AIDS not donate blood."

And what did that standard of care require the Red Cross or other blood banks to do during that time period?

"Screening out of donors at risk of acquiring the AIDS agent; orally educating the donor regarding their risk; giving the written materials is also desirable. And then actually finding out if the donor understands the risk of transmitting AIDS, and if they are involved in those behaviors, how they can easily defer from donating blood."

Would a blood bank such as the Red Cross have to implement those steps in order to meet the standard of care? Feldman asked.

"I think so, yes."

"Did the Red Cross implement any of these methods that you suggested as of July 1984, a year and a half after the January meeting, at the time that the blood was donated that was ultimately transfused into Roland Ray?"

"Only the pamphlets," Francis replied.

The Red Cross's response to the meeting and a subsequent FDA recommendation had been, Francis said, a passive approach: "self-deferral." The Red Cross did not orally inform blood donors about AIDS or the high-risk groups, and it did not ask donors confidential questions about high-risk behaviors. Instead, the Red Cross gave all donors a modified copy of a pamphlet it had been using for years entitled, "What You Should Know about Giving Blood." The cover of the pamphlet did not indicate the importance of the information inside, or the addition of new information on AIDS. A blood donor, who was assumed to be literate, was expected, based on his reading of the pamphlet, to identify himself as a high-risk donor, recognize the implications of giving blood, and decline to donate.

"Did the Red Cross's use only of the pamphlets in July of 1984 constitute, in your opinion, what a reasonable and prudent blood banker should have done by that date?" Feldman asked.

"No," Francis said. "I think handing out pamphlets has traditionally been one of the weakest forms of health education."

"Do you have an opinion when the scientific community, including the blood banking community, had enough information to be reasonably certain that AIDS was transmissible by blood?"

"I certainly do. At the January meeting there was plenty of information available, in 1983."

Feldman offered Plaintiff's Exhibit 19, a letter to Arnie deBeaufort from Joseph P. O'Malley, head of the Red Cross Office of Product Development. The letter was dated February 1, 1983. Francis told the jury, "It says very clearly that AIDS is transmissible by blood."

"Did the Public Health Service of the federal government ever recommend that high-risk donors be excluded?"

"Yes," Francis replied. "In March 1983, a month after this letter."

Supporting Francis's statement, Feldman produced a letter from Dennis Donohue, FDA's blood chief to Fred Katz, dated March 15, 1983. Francis explained that the letter directed blood collectors to implement procedures to educate donors about AIDS and AIDS risk groups. It further told them to develop procedures to screen high-risk individuals, including sexually active gay men. FDA also recommended that studies of donor screening procedures be undertaken to determine the most effective method for screening those at high risk of AIDS.

The industry's Joint Statement of January 13, 1983 then came before the court. After several objections by Red Cross counsel, Francis read aloud a highlighted paragraph: "There is currently considerable pressure on the blood banking community to restrict blood donations from gay males. Direct or indirect questions about a donor's sexual preference are inappropriate. Such an invasion can be justified only if it demonstrates a clear-cut benefit. In fact, there is reason to believe that such questions, no matter how well intentioned, are ineffective in eliminating those donors who may carry AIDS."

In Francis's opinion, that statement, coming nine days after the CDC meeting, was an overt rejection of federal recommendations regarding the screening of blood and donors.

"Doctor, in your opinion, if a blood bank refused to implement direct questioning by July 1984, and blood was collected that was transfused into Mr. Ray, had they deviated from the standard of care and failed to act in a reasonably and prudent manner to protect the blood supply?"

"Absolutely," Francis said.

If, in 1984, a blood bank did not conduct donor questioning in a confidential setting, would that also violate the standard of care, and if it did not inform donors of high-risk groups, would that, too, be in violation?

To both questions, Francis responded, "Yes, it would. As articulated by the FDA, blood banks were told to inform donors, as part of the screening procedures, who was at risk, and so, yes, it is below the standard of care not to do that."

As for the "cafeteria-like" setting in which Roland Ray's donor gave blood, would that environment, Feldman asked, deviate from the standard of care as defined by what a reasonable and prudent blood bank would do? Francis said it would be a violation of the standard, "not to mention pure logic."

Feldman produced several letters from Dr. Pearl Toy, director of the San Jose region of the Red Cross. Peter Bleakley objected and continued to enter objections as Feldman asked Francis about Toy's letters. In June 1983, Toy had directed her staff to be certain that the donors had read and understood the AIDS information. The document also indicated, Francis told the jury, that donors were not reading the Red Cross pamphlet. By June 1984, San Jose had broken ranks with headquarters by quizzing donors about the contents of the pamphlets and instituting surrogate testing. San Jose had reported seventeen cases of AIDS in 1984. For that same period, in Washington D.C., which conducted no such direct donor questioning, eighty-five cases of AIDS had been reported.

"Do you have an opinion, within a reasonable degree of certainty, as to whether or not the donor screening practice in the District of Columbia region of the American Red Cross as of July of 1984 deviated from the standard of care?"

"As defined as what would be reasonable and prudent for a blood bank? They did not act reasonably and prudently."

Feldman asked whether the Red Cross followed FDA recommendations about educating donors. Francis replied it did not. Did the Red Cross undertake studies as prescribed by FDA to determine the efficacy of donor screening to eliminate gay men? No, Francis said, it did not.

Peter Bleakley's cross-examination returned to Francis's lack of direct involvement in blood banking. Wasn't Francis speaking as someone from CDC when he said Red Cross was not complying with FDA recommendations? Yes, Francis said, he was. Didn't Francis know, in fact, that FDA officials had not expressed opinions that the Red Cross did not comply with their recommendations? No, Francis said, he did not know that for a fact, but he presumed FDA believed the Red Cross was complying with its recommendations.

As for his statement that the Red Cross failed in its AIDS education efforts, Bleakley pointed out, "In fact, the American Red Cross right here in Washington, D.C. attempted to educate the community about the risk of AIDS and who was at high risk."

Francis replied, "I would not be surprised if they did try."

And, didn't he also know for a fact that the Red Cross had met with gay groups in D.C. to discuss screening measures? Francis said he had read something to that effect. And didn't he know, for a fact, that the Red Cross had a call-back procedure by which high-risk donors would defer that donation? Francis said he thought that was a good idea, if it were delivered properly so that the donor understood.

Bleakley referred to CDC's summary report of the January 4, 1983 meeting. There had been no consensus reached at that meeting as to direct questioning, wasn't that right? Francis said, "I think we covered that this morning, yes." Bleakley read from that summary, which cited the advantage of direct donor questioning as "an easy extension of the screening history, but having the disadvantage of being potentially intrusive."

Francis said, "I think it's worthwhile hearing the last sentence," which he then read aloud: "Some commercial plasmapherisis processes are already excluding by history some AIDS high-risk groups."

Bleakley returned to CDC's summary, and the lack of consensus on direct donor questioning. Francis explained, "That wasn't the purpose of the document. FDA, CDC and NIH all recommended direct questioning. The recommendations were clearly made and put on the back of the blood collecting industry to evaluate and, indeed, at the January meeting the blood banks agreed to do that."

About the joint statement, Bleakley asked, didn't Francis know, in fact, that FDA had approved the document? Francis said he did not know that for a fact, but that he would not be surprised if FDA had. "These are individuals with no experience dealing with direct questioning of gay men who made that decision," Francis said.

Bleakley cited various Red Cross studies of direct questioning, to which Francis countered, "There was no rigorous evaluation. The purpose and the consensus was that men at risk, especially gay and bisexual men, should be screened from blood donating systems. There was no evaluation for that. The reality was, no one went in and did the simple questioning, asking people walking in the door about their sexual orientation."

Bleakley concluded his cross-examination of Dr. Francis by pointing out that he was a paid expert witness who earned, in 1992, in excess of $70,000 as a witness.

On redirect, Feldman asked Francis, "Do you do this for the money?"

Francis said he did not.

Why, then?

"I ask myself that frequently when I sit up on stands like this," Francis replied. "My interest was stimulated by the testimony I saw from Red Cross officials about what CDC was saying, and thought that should be corrected."

Feldman's next witness was the San Francisco AIDS specialist Dr. Marcus Conant. The two had met at the July 1990 hearings of John Dingell's Subcommittee on Oversight and Investigations of the House Committee on Energy and Commerce. Conant had then testified that FDA and Red Cross had a symbiotic relationship. Now, at the Roland Ray trial, Conant said that the Red Cross had failed to meet FDA recommendations; that it had adequate information about blood-borne AIDS, but had not taken appropriate action. Conant attempted to elucidate the relationship between the regulators and the Red Cross.

Peter Bleakley objected, "I know this man has alleged since 1987 in testimony that he thinks they [Red Cross and FDA] were in bed together, that there was a massive conspiracy. I'm worried about it being improper, that we would get one of his speeches."

Feldman decided to take another tack. He went to the core of the standard of care issue. "Does the fact," he asked Conant, "that many of the blood banks were doing the same thing as the Red Cross, does that mean in your opinion, to a reasonable degree of certainty, that the Red Cross had met the standard?"

"No, sir," Conant replied. "An industry can be negligent and the fact that the whole industry was doing the wrong thing doesn't mean that part of that industry is okay because they were doing the same thing that everybody else was doing. The entire industry fell below a reasonable standard to exclude all members of high-risk groups."

Under questioning by Bleakley, Conant testified that in 1987, he became involved in AIDS cases. Only then did he realize that the Red Cross had not been asking crucial questions in 1984. "I was then of the opinion that they did fall below the standard of care, because they didn't do what the FDA told them to do."

Bleakley asked, "You are not an expert on interpreting FDA regulations, are you, sir?"

"I didn't know there was a specialty in interpreting Food and Drug regulations, sir. They speak for themselves."

Bleakley continued to challenge Conant. Conant did not know whether FDA agreed with his assessment, wasn't that correct? Conant said that was correct; he did not know. And didn't Conant know that Red Cross had made an effort to educate the public? "I'm sure the Red Cross did put on a few programs for physicians," the doctor replied. "But they did not have an effective program to educate the public." Conant specifically cited his review of the deposition of Dr. Gerald Sandler, associate director of Blood Services. He told the court that when Sandler was asked about Red Cross's educational efforts, he had stated, "That was not our responsibility."

It was indeed the responsibility of the Red Cross, Conant said, and FDA had made that clear.

"Isn't it a fact, Dr. Conant," Bleakley went on, "that the screening measures that were put in place in 1983 by the American Red Cross and other blood banks throughout the United States were effective in significantly reducing the number of high-risk donors giving blood?"

"No, sir. I do not accept that for one moment. Not only were they not effective in reducing the number of high-risk donors, they failed in their obligation to protect donors by not helping stop the spread of the AIDS epidemic."

As witnesses took the stand, and the attorneys skirmished over admissibility of evidence. Roland Ray sat with his wife, Janet, and listened. It had been eleven years since his blood transfusion. His T-cell count had fluctuated but was now stable. He had had a few bad bouts, which AZT seemed to make worse. He had told his doctor, Fred Gill, that he did not want to continue taking the drug. He did not want his family to see him become so debilitated, not before it was his time. He already had to quit work and live more quietly, which had been difficult. He was a working man. He had managed to find projects to do at home—cultivating a garden, building pens for Emily's goats and rabbits. And he had begun planning an addition to the house which he hoped, over time, to build with his father's help.

He was remarkably alive. For whatever reason, he was defying the odds.

From time to time, Roland looked behind him and saw his mother and one of his sisters. But not his dad. It hurt his father to even speak the word "AIDS." Every night Harry Ray wanted to know what had transpired in court, but he could not bring himself to attend. Harry Ray was from the old school: if you didn't talk about it, maybe it would be all right.

Roland was glad his father had not heard much of the testimony, particularly when Fred Gill had taken the stand. Peter Vangsnes had assumed the questioning. He asked Dr. Gill to tell the court about Roland Ray's health history, the effects of AZT, the emotional toll on the Ray family. Fred Gill was a deeply compassionate man, and he had been reluctant to discuss Ray's prognosis, with Roland's mother and wife in court. But Vangsnes persisted, and Gill had answered truthfully.

"I believe," Dr. Gill said, "that he is going to die from this infection, that he is going to develop AIDS, and he will get either one of the bad infections that are known as opportunistic infections or one of the severe complications of AIDS, and that at the present time we can delay this, but we can't stop it from happening."

It had been upsetting, as well, hearing for the first time the donor's testimony as it played in court. Over the years, Roland had wondered about this man whose blood would kill him. Listening to the tape on the second day of the trial, he felt no anger. "Mr. Donor" was a man with a wife and family. His being bisexual and barely literate did not make him a bad man. He had simply been misinformed.

At trial, Roland learned that Dr. Alfred Katz, head of Blood Services, had known there was a crisis long before his transfusion. Katz had been deposed by Chris Tisi and an excerpt of that deposition had been read into the trial record.

TISI: Did there come a time in your mind when it was probable or very likely that AIDS can be transmitted by blood or blood products?

KATZ: I think by late 1983.

TISI: What caused you to come to that conclusion in late 1983?

KATZ: To come to the probability as we had discussed it previously, the accumulation of information coming from CDC associated with patients who developed AIDS who had transfusions from high-risk donors.

TISI: Were there any particular articles, publications, that would have helped you come to this conclusion?

KATZ: Publications of CDC that appeared in the *New England Journal of Medicine* in January 1984.

TISI: Did you believe that there was a percentage of individuals that were not voluntarily removing themselves based upon the pamphlet and the questions that were being asked of that person?

KATZ: For a variety of reasons.

TISI: It was likely that a certain percentage were continuing to donate?

KATZ: That should not have been.

TISI: Did you presume that was likely in January 1984?

KATZ: Yes.

What Roland Ray found incredible was that the Red Cross could actually have stopped the spread of AIDS through blood. Why hadn't it?

It made no sense to him, no sense at all.

But of all the testimony, the most difficult for him was Janet's. It was not what she said, it was her having to say it in front of strangers. She had to expose the details of their marriage, her most intimate thoughts and feelings, and he was unable to protect her. He tried to hold back during his own testimony, tried to keep some things private. But then he began talking about the baby, Emily, how she would imitate his magic trick, to try to make him well again. "Here, Daddy," she'd say, "I'll do magic and make you better." Even as he spoke those words, he broke down.

Later that day, he almost lost it again. As court was adjourned for the night, he watched several Red Cross attorneys walking to the elevator. They were laughing. Roland wanted to go up to them and shout, "This is my life, my *life*. This is not some game."

Janet must have known, because she held him back until the attorneys headed downstairs, where chauffeured cars awaited.

On May 10, Peter Bleakley's associate Fern O'Brian asked the judge to take the Roland Ray case out of the jury's hands. She requested a directed verdict—that Salzman himself render a decision. O'Brian argued that Ray's attorneys "have failed to provide any objective, factual basis for the standard of care, that the standard of care includes measures that the experts claim the Red Cross should have adopted, including direct oral questioning of donors about sexual practices."

She said his attorneys had provided no evidence and no testimony that any other blood bank or plasma collecting organization was conducting such measures as of July 1984. They had provided no evidence that any government agency required, recommended or even advised such measures be adopted. And they provided no evidence that any study showed such measures would have been effective.

Salzman told O'Brian, "Surely there is evidence, is there not, Ms. O'Brian, that the types of screening procedures used by the Red Cross were inappropriate because they didn't provide sufficient privacy and direct requests? In other words, if I may use a crude analogy, one who is required by the rules of the road to look must look effectively. One who is required by regulations or inspection must screen effectively in light of what he knows. It is no help if they ask questions when it is not likely the answers will be given satisfactorily, ma'am.

"It doesn't take an enormous scientific study to know, I would suggest to you, madam, within the common sense of jurors, if they choose to believe it, that the type of personal questions asked in the presence of one's co-workers which were normally private is something that you may not get a candid response to if you haven't provided a closed setting."

Salzman concluded, "There is certainly evidence on the record from two people who appeared to be qualified or could be found to be qualified by the jurors, if they wish, that the Red Cross should have used a more direct, private, and pointed type of screening than they did. That the type of screening they used generally and in this case in particular was very likely to be ineffective. I am satisfied that a reasonable juror could find that there was an appropriate standard of care established, that the standard of care was not met by the Red Cross, and that its failure to meet the standard of care was the approximate cause of the injury."

The judge denied the Red Cross's motion for a directed verdict.

Mike Feldman was looking forward to questioning Dr. Gerald Sandler. As associate director of Blood Services for the Red Cross from 1978 through 1984, Jerry Sandler's advice was frequently sought in connection with the AIDS issue. Feldman had made notes of some of the key issues while the Red Cross was examining its first witness, Dr. Thomas Zuck. Zuck was professor of Transfusion Medicine at the Hocksworth Blood Center of the University of Cincinnati Medical Center. He supported the Red Cross's claim that its existing screening mechanisms were "highly effective in terms of reducing the people that we did not want to give blood, that is, those people who engaged in risky behavior." Zuck testified that in 1983 it had come to the attention of the blood banking community that AIDS might be blood borne. As a result, the Red Cross amended its donor registration card. The additional questions on the card concerned signs and symptoms of AIDS.

Zuck also pointed to two studies the Red Cross had conducted, one in Penn-Jersey, the other in Atlanta. Those studies showed that direct questioning of male donors reduced donations by between three and ten percent.

Feldman intended to dispel any notions the jury had that the Red Cross had conducted studies that were not self-serving. It was through Gerald Sandler that he intended to prove the Red Cross's negligence.

Fern O'Brian began questioning Sandler on behalf of the Red Cross. Sandler told the jury that the Red Cross had initiated a callback system. Donors could inform the collection centers that their blood should not be used. "We also were very eager to distribute Public Health Service facts about AIDS and make sure that all of our blood centers had the very latest documents," Sandler said. "The most obvious change was when we made a change in the pamphlet, it is to totally redesign the pamphlet, so that if you are a regular blood donor and you see a pamphlet that sort of lies horizontally, it says the Red Cross this way, and it's mostly red, and then the next one you are going to see is when we make a change, [it] is going to be a vertical one and it's going to be mostly white and black, or something to that effect. So you know there's been a change and you know to focus your attention on it."

Sandler told the court that a directive issued on June 1984 had revised the "entire process of collecting blood and managing blood. [It] asked about any recent onset of signs and symptoms of AIDS."

Sandler told the jury that research was conducted at several regions. "It was really quite difficult to do any research to find out if someone had the capability of transmitting AIDS by blood if there was no test, and at that time there was no way to measure the virus. There was nothing that you could really do to measure this." Reiterating Dr. Zuck's testimony, Sandler explained that the Red Cross had conducted studies in Cleveland, Philadelphia, and Atlanta. These studies showed that the Red Cross's self-deferral system was effective.

When asked about his decision to reject direct donor questioning, Sandler explained, "People that I respected who were gay, who were physicians, who were government officials, had said to me . . . don't ask direct questions, it's not going to work, and you're going to get just the opposite effect."

On Tuesday morning, May 11, Feldman began his cross-examination of Jerry Sandler. Just as Bleakley had challenged Don Francis's qualifications in blood banking, Feldman challenged Sandler's knowledge of epidemiology, virology, and infectious disease. Sandler was certified in none of those specialties.

The prior day, Sandler had discussed the Red Cross's operations. Feldman now asked him for more detail. Wasn't it true that the Red Cross collected blood from volunteer donors and sold that blood to hospital or transfusion services?

"Not true," Sandler said.

"Isn't it true that they receive a fee for providing the blood to hospitals or transfusion services?"

"Yes."

And isn't it true that fee goes to more than covering the cost of the collection process; that is, there are excesses over revenues?

"No," Sandler said.

Sandler's answer was curious in light of the Red Cross's own financial reports. In 1993, Blood Services had earned the Red Cross $955.8 million.

Feldman asked Sandler whether he had concerns, in 1983, that high-risk donors were not self deferring, that they were "getting through the screening procedures."

Sandler said he did.

"And isn't it true that by July of 1984, it was known to you that homosexual or bisexual men with multiple partners were probably continuing to donate blood?"

"Some," Sandler said.

"And, in fact, you knew by July of 1984 that the pamphlet in question wasn't working in the D.C. area, isn't that true?"

"No."

"Isn't it true," Feldman asked, "that as of July of 1984 in the D.C. region of the American Red Cross, you knew there were donors who had been given the pamphlet and were asked to self-defer and were higher-risk and still giving blood?"

"I assumed that to be true," Sandler said.

Didn't he know it for a fact to be true?

"I don't think I knew it as a fact, but I assumed it to be true and acted as though I did know it. But I can't point to knowing it."

"Did you assume," Feldman asked, "that there could be people in the blood donor pool that were, in fact, illiterate or could not read or fully understand the pamphlet?"

Yes, he did. He expected donors to say that they had not read and understood the pamphlet.

"And wouldn't it have been a check on the ability, the effectiveness of the question 'Did you read and understand?' to know if the percentage of the people answering no equated somewhat with the percentage of the people who were illiterate in a particular population?"

"No." Sandler said. He said that eighty-five percent of the donors had been through the system at least once before. "And we assumed a certain level of comprehension of the process."

But did he know whether those repeat donors were literate or illiterate, just by the fact that they were repeat donors?

"Other than by the definitions we've talked about, no," Sandler replied. "We wanted this in the way the FDA wanted it, as fast as we could possibly do it, and not delay by doing some study forehand."

Feldman showed Dr. Sandler Plaintiff's Exhibit 187: the May 23,

1984 minutes of the Medical Advisory Committee meeting in Syracuse, New York. Dr. Harold Lamberson was medical director of that region. "He would have been number one or probably number two," Sandler said of Lamberson's position.

Sandler read aloud, "Dr. Lamberson announced that the National Red Cross does have access to the test and has tested one thousand, five hundred samples from the Washington, D.C. center. They have, in fact, found some positive donors whose units have been transfused."

Feldman asked, "Now isn't it true, Doctor, that out of one thousand five hundred hundred samples in March of 1984, that there were some of those one thousand five hundred samples that were found to be HIV positive as a result of a prelicensed test?"

"Not necessarily," Sandler replied.

"What is meant by 'they have found some positive donors whose units have been transfused'?"

"What is meant is that we had agreed to cooperate with Dr. Robert Gallo at NIH to look at the validity of an experimental research test that he had, and he was testing the validity of his test against some people in the blood donor population to find out how many reactors there would be. Whether these were positive or not was the question he was asking us, not we were asking him."

"Doctor, isn't this evidence of the fact that high-risk people in the blood donor pool were still giving blood in the D.C. region?"

"Not those two sentences."

"Thank you, Doctor. You knew in 1983 and 1984 that there were donors who were infected but who showed no signs or symptoms of AIDS, correct?"

Sandler said that was correct. And yes, he knew that the incubation period was about two years.

"As of July of 1984, when Roland Ray's donor gave blood you had no doubt in your mind, Doctor, isn't it true, that AIDS could be transmitted by blood transfusion?"

"No doubt."

Feldman showed Sandler the Red Cross pamphlet. He asked him to read the first sentence.

"The newly described illness of unknown cause is believed to be spread by intimate personal contact and possibly by blood transfusions."

"Doctor, this was used in July of 1984?"

"Yes," it was.

"And that's not a true statement, is it, Doctor?"

"It's not as precise as we want it."

"It is inaccurate information to tell a donor in July of 1984, is it not, that AIDS is possibly spread by blood transfusion, when in fact you knew it it was spread by blood transfusion, correct?"

"That's not correct."

Did he believe that there was any doubt that AIDS was transmitted by blood as of July of 1984?

Sandler said, "I think we're dealing with just a tiny difference between us. I had a small doubt, and there were many people out there who had a big doubt. But I think you and I are very close. I was very close to complete belief but retained a slight doubt."

"What's the difference between slight doubt and a moment ago when you told me there was no doubt?"

"That's pretty obvious to me."

"I think so, too, Doctor. Would you admit, Doctor, that by March of '83, when the Public Health Service and the FDA issued its recommendations regarding eliminating the high-risk groups, you believed that the Red Cross should proceed on the assumption that AIDS was transmissible by blood transfusion?"

"True."

"And did you believe that as of March of 1983 that the Red Cross should take all reasonable steps to eliminate those identified at high risk of contracting AIDS from the blood donor pool?"

"No."

"Why not?"

"Your definition would include all gay persons. The Public Health Service advised us and the FDA required us to use a different definition than the one that appears here, which is specifically 'sexually active homosexual or bisexual men with multiple partners.' And the difference is between the larger group and the smaller group, and that's why I answered as I did."

Feldman rephrased the question. "Would you agree that the Red Cross, as of March of 1983, should have taken all reasonable steps to eliminate from the blood donor pool those defined by the FDA as being high risk for contracting AIDS?"

"If you mean persons identified at increased risk of developing AIDS—that's a specific definition—yes."

"So whether or not you personally believed that AIDS was transmissible by blood or not in March of 1983, you proceeded as if it was, correct?"

"Yes."

Feldman referred Sandler back to the prior day's testimony regarding potential blood shortages. "So it is your testimony that if you eliminated all gay men from the blood donor pool in 1983, you would not have been able to meet the blood transfusion needs of the United States?"

"Yes," Sandler said, "but not because of the loss of the relatively few units of blood, but because of the broader consequences that would have involved such a controversial policy."

Was it feasible, Feldman asked, to restrict all gay men from the blood donor pool in 1983?

Sandler said, yes, it was.

Feldman questioned Sandler about his belief that high-risk donors should be excluded from blood donation. He referenced Sandler's article published in the Israeli *Journal of Medical Science* in 1975, which discussed hepatitis B and high-risk donors. Wasn't it true, Feldman asked, that in 1975, in the U.S., gay and bisexual men's behavior put them at higher risk for hepatitis B than the general population?

Sandler replied, "Yes, in 1975 that was probably true."

Wasn't it true that the Red Cross could ask direct question of donors without receiving FDA approval?

"Not true," Sandler said.

Feldman referred to a letter already in exhibit from the Penn-Jersey region. That center had initiated direct question of donors in 1983. Sandler was asked to read aloud from the staff directive: "We will ask: 'Do you fit into any of the high-risk groups as described 'In an Important Message' to all donors using a question."

Wasn't that a direct question?

"It is a direct question that refers to sexual preference."

Had that been approved by the FDA?

Sandler said, "This was a research pilot study that I approved at national headquarters within the variance that would be allowable. To the best of my knowledge, this may also have been known to the FDA as a research study."

"Isn't it true, Doctor, that without seeking FDA approval, a region of the American Red Cross would be permitted to quiz donors about their knowledge of who was a high risk for AIDS in order to ensure that the pamphlets were being read?"

"I don't believe so."

Feldman referred to the April 23, 1984 letter from the San Jose region of the Red Cross, indicating that San Jose was ensuring donors were reading the pamphlet by asking them to identify the four high-risk groups.

Sandler responded, "I don't know the context that this was written, and it's possible that the block—again, we're dealing with things that are ten years ago. But there is a block or an empty square where you could fill in the question. It's possible that this responds to that. It's also possible that this is part of some pilot study that I don't recall, or it's possible that they did this."

"Had FDA approved that, yes or no?"

"I don't know. I don't recall that event."

"Could a Red Cross region have implemented such a program without FDA approval?"

"In a limited sense as you described, yes."

"Wasn't this blood bank in San Jose and other non–Red Cross blood banks taking steps to eliminate high-risk donors?"

"Yes."

Feldman then returned to the literacy issue.

"Now, if some donors were not reading the pamphlet, then those donors were not being informed of the high-risk groups at the donation site."

"Probably," Sandler said.

"And if a blood bank knew that donors weren't reading the pamphlet, then that blood bank knew that the donors were not being informed of who was at high risk for AIDS at the donation site, correct?"

"If all of your ifs pertain to Washington, the answer is yes," Sandler said.

"If a blood bank knew that donors were not being informed of high-risk groups for AIDS, the blood bank was not following FDA recommendations, correct?"

"Yes."

"And FDA required that donors be informed, whether or not they could read the pamphlet?" Feldman asked.

"Sure."

"And didn't the Red Cross know, prior to July 1984, that all donors were not reading the pamphlet?"

"We presumed that there were some donors that weren't reading the pamphlet. That's a fair statement." But, he said, he "had no knowledge that some people who weren't reading the book were also some people at high risk."

"Well, you knew that high-risk donors were continuing to donate, though, didn't you, Doctor, as of July of 1984?"

"Yes."

"Would orally informing donors, reading them the high-risk groups that were in the pamphlet, not asking them anything, would that have ensured that people who couldn't read were getting the information that you wanted to get to them?"

"No."

"Why not?"

"Oh, we all listen to an awful lot of things when people talk to us when it goes by. And if it's technical, we don't all catch it. Under some circumstances you don't get a chance to ask questions about clarification."

"No harm in doing both, though, is there, doctor?" Feldman said.

Sandler replied, "As long as we don't measure harm in discouraging blood donors and creating an environment where people don't give blood, there's probably no harm being done. But I got a hunch if I read out everything that's in this pamphlet to each and every person each and every time they came, some people might have found the process one that they would not want to go through. I don't know. I never test that."

"You never studied that, correct?" Feldman asked.

"Never studied it."

CHAPTER FIFTEEN

FALL FROM GRACE

May 1993–December 1993

There was a sense of chaos, a fair amount of panic and paranoia. People were running scared.

Former Midwest Regional Officer
The American Red Cross

It was the office of a powerful woman who seemed to have everything under control—immense in proportion, with high ceilings, conservative, neutral colors, nothing striking or particularly personal about it. There were several original oil paintings of historic value, photos of Elizabeth Dole, smiling, with world leaders, photos of a much younger Bob Dole. A fireplace that was rarely lit. Large windows overlooked the Mall, the grassy esplanade that extended from the Washington Monument to the Capitol, bordered by the stately colonnades of national museums and art galleries.

Looking eastward from her second-story window, Mrs. Dole had an unobstructed view of the White House.

The Marble Palace, Red Cross's national headquarters, was completed in February, 1917, on a site which had been given, in perpetuity, to the Red Cross by the U.S. government. At the groundbreaking ceremony two years earlier, President Taft dedicated the building to the memory of the heroic women of the Civil War, "that their labors to mitigate the sufferings of the sick and wounded in the war may be perpetuated."

The cost of the imposing structure—$800,000, was paid in part by congressional appropriation, the rest by private benefactors, including Mrs. Russell Sage, Mrs. E. H. Harriman and the Rockefeller

Foundation. Its palatial trappings would reflect its stature. Ornate double staircases, a cavernous marble grand hall. Stained windows commissioned from the Tiffany Studios in New York depicted Red Cross women, their ministry through sacrifice.

It was here that presidents and princesses would pay homage to the legacy of Clara Barton.

On this mild morning in May 1993, as testimony continued in Roland Ray's case, the mood within the Marble Palace was less than exalted. Indeed, among those gathered in Mrs. Dole's office, the tenor bordered on hysteria. They were all there, the Special Team as well as high-level Red Cross staff—which in itself was unusual. The Special Team generally met sequestered from the staff. But today the group was integrated. There was Karen Shoos Lipton, Red Cross general counsel; Fred Kyle, executive vice president of Blood Services; Peter Tomasulo, head of Blood Services operations; John Heubusch, communications director; Michael Goldfarb, Blood Services consultant; and, of course, Jenna Dorn and Mari Maseng-Will. Today, the usual in-fighting to gain Mrs. Dole's attention and favor had an edge.

Names were bandied about, high-level officials who might be called on to call off FDA and the Department of Justice. John Dingell, for one.

"Elizabeth, talk to him, nobody can tell the story better than you," a member of her Special Team prompted.

Mrs. Dole was reminded to call Donna Shalala. The secretary of Health and Human Services would need to be told that the Red Cross blood was safe.

Elizabeth Dole sat quietly for long periods of time, saying nothing. She looked from face to face, as if she were watching a tennis match and hadn't a clue as to how the game was played. She knew only that her survival depended on who won.

This was a crisis of unprecedented proportion. On May 7, the U.S. Department of Justice on behalf of FDA had formally filed a "Complaint for Permanent Injunction" against the American Red Cross. The thirty-two-page document, which included a Consent Decree, had been faxed to the corporate counsel's office in early April. The serious federal charges had been brought under the Federal Food, Drug and Cosmetic [FD&C] Act, 21 U.S.C. 332(a) and the District Court of Washington D.C.'s "inherent equity power." The court was being asked to order the Red Cross to cease from manufacturing, processing, shipping, and delivering "adulterated" and "misbranded" blood and blood products.

The FDA was requesting that the Red Cross be put under permanent injunction. Only through this directive, FDA told the courts, could the Red Cross be prevented from issuing dangerous blood and blood product.

United States of America v. American National Red Cross, Civil no. 93 0949, charged the Red Cross with "introducing or delivering for introduction into interstate commerce drugs that are . . . (i) adulterated . . . that the methods used to manufacture, process, pack, or hold the drugs do not conform to current good manufacturing practice; to assure that such drugs meet the requirements . . . as to safety, identity, strength, quality, and purity; and (ii) misbranded . . ."

It also charged the Red Cross with violating regulations of the Public Health Service Act "which establish standards designed to prevent the introduction, transmission, or spread of communicable diseases from foreign countries into the United States and from one state to another state . . ."

"Because blood products are living tissue," the complaint stated, "use of these products can present both life-supporting and life-threatening situations. Accordingly, it is crucial that the process by which blood and blood components are manufactured, processed, packed, held, and labeled are rigorously controlled."

The Red Cross's more recent history of violating federal blood safety laws was summarized. Between April 1990 and February 1993, FDA inspections of Red Cross headquarters and centers "revealed continuing violations of the Food, Drug and Cosmetic Act, the PHS Act, and the regulations relating to blood products." FDA had issued "notices of intent" to revoke licenses for the Albany, New York region in 1989 and the Charleston, South Carolina and Portland, Oregon regions in 1991, and it had revoked those licenses. "Despite having been warned that the conditions at its facilities might subject the ARC to regulatory action, and notwithstanding the 1988 agreement, the violations persist."

The petition for permanent injunction cited FDA's inspections of several Red Cross regions which "documented" violations of current good manufacturing practice and biological product regulations in the manufacture of blood products." As a result of these and other deviations, the Red Cross signed an agreement with FDA on September 14, 1988, in which it agreed to establish clear lines of control between national headquarters and regions to improve training and auditing and to review and redesign computer systems to ensure that unsuitable blood products were not released or transfused.

Yet according to the FDA complaint, there were still deviations in the manufacture, processing, packing, and holding of blood products. Red Cross officials had been formally advised of the violations at the end of each inspection. Although the Red Cross had made changes to its operations (it shut down one region and underwent a major reorganization), it continued to commit violations of the Federal Food, Drug and Cosmetic Act, the Public Health Service Act, and applicable regulations.

So recalcitrant was the Red Cross that, FDA concluded, "unless the court grants the relief sought in this complaint, the ARC may continue to violate" the applicable laws "in the manner alleged."

FDA had essentially thrown up its hands. Only by permanently enjoining "the Red Cross and each of its officers, agents, representatives, employees, attorneys, and all persons in active concert or participation with them" could it hope to stop the organization from issuing contaminated blood. It further asked the court to enjoin the Red Cross to establish clear lines of managerial control over quality assurance and quality control in all regions; establish and implement a comprehensive quality assurance/quality control program; and establish and implement a comprehensive training program to ensure that all personnel engaged in the manufacture, processing, packing, holding, and distribution of blood products were adequate in number and qualified to perform their duties.

During her prior years in government, Elizabeth Dole had managed to stay one step ahead of congressional mandate by announcing some kind of reformation. She had done as much in 1991, by proposing Transformation. But this time there was no quick fix. "The 'Let's pull another one out of our hats' maneuver which was standard operating procedure with Elizabeth was not going to work this time," recalled one official involved in those crisis meetings.

The petition for permanent injunction was scheduled to be heard May 12.

Potential avenues of redress were quickly exhausted. None of Mrs. Dole's powerful Capitol Hill connections interceded in federal court. The Red Cross could counter the charges, vigorously contest the Department of Justice's allegations, and proceed to court, but that would mean a rather embarrassing public exposure of its policies. On the other hand, it could sign the Consent Decree, agreeing to abide by the terms of the complaint.

Mrs. Dole was reluctant to sign the Consent Decree.

Kyle, Peter Tomasulo, and general counsel Karen Shoos Lipton worked with Arnold & Porter, some of whose other clients had faced regulatory ire. Their task was to deliver a "benign Consent Decree."

Several incarnations later, an alternate Decree had been hashed out by representatives of the Red Cross. The Decree no longer referred to Elizabeth Dole by name. The Red Cross agreed to operate under the permanent injunction without admitting to any of the charges. It would be required to meet specified timetables for improving blood safety at its forty-seven regional blood centers, including ensuring quality control, training, and data management. Unlike in the voluntary agreement, the Red Cross was required to abide by the terms of the Decree or face potential criminal sanctions, including contempt. If it remained in serious violation, it could go into receivership. Theoretically, FDA could assume control over a large part of the Red Cross's operations. Such action was considered unlikely, since the FDA lacked the resources to manage the largest blood collector in the nation.

The Red Cross would also be responsible for reimbursing the FDA for the costs of all government inspections and examinations necessary to evaluate compliance with the Consent Decree. That meant the Red Cross would have to pay the FDA $47 an hour for inspections; $56.50 an hour for analytical work; 25 cents a mile for travel expenses; and as much as $147 a day for "subsistence expenses," when necessary. The total reimbursement was not to exceed $250,000 per year. If the Red Cross violated any of the Consent Decree stipulations and was found in civil or criminal contempt, it would be required to reimburse FDA and the Justice Department for attorney fees and other costs relating to any proceedings.

Five years from entry of the Consent Decree, the Red Cross could petition for relief, a request that its status be reviewed. But if there were significant failures to comply with the law or with the Consent Decree, FDA could deny its request.

The court retained jurisdiction over this action for the purpose of enforcing and modifying this decree, and for granting such additional relief as might be necessary or appropriate.

But there was a catch, a loophole through which violations like issuing HIV-infected blood could slip. The Consent Decree stipulated that "the FDA shall not base its decision whether to take enforcement action under this decree based solely upon the number of FD-483 observations [inspection reports] or the number of recalls."

Elizabeth Dole subsequently assured the public, "This agreement will help strengthen the safety redundancies and guarantees already built into the system."

To those who were familiar with Mrs. Dole's management style, the federal injunction came as no surprise. It had become apparent to John Dingell's staff director, Steve Sims, that when she had announced Transformation, there had been no plan. "It didn't exist," Sims said. "It was a PR attempt to try to put the Red Cross in the best light. It didn't fool FDA. It took off the political heat, but in point of fact, things were not getting better."

What he did find extraordinary was the absence of Mrs. Dole's name on the Consent Decree. "When a consent decree comes down, what does it contain? It contains the conditions you have to comply with, and the name of the president of the organization. Every lawyer has said this is a very unusual consent decree."

It seemed to Sims that Mrs. Dole had walked into a bad situation and made it worse. Yet somehow, she had gotten off the hook.

Dr. David Jenkins, director of Red Cross's Louisville region, commented, "It's criminal, what they let her get away with."

On the morning of May 17, Judge Richard Salzman discussed with counsels the instructions he planned to give the jury. The purpose of such instruction was not to tell the jury what they could find, but how to go about arriving at their decision. Since the Ray case pivoted on the issue of standard of care, each side had submitted in writing its own definition to the judge. As expected, there was much disagreement. Arnold & Porter counsel Fern O'Brian argued that the Red Cross should be judged according to the standard of care applicable to other professions. Ashcraft & Gerel's Peter Vangsnes said that the standard should be based on what actions were prudent and reasonable.

Judge Salzman finally directed the jury that "The standard of care is defined as follows: They must use the degree of skill, care, and learning ordinarily possessed and used by others practicing in their field in the same or similar circumstances. Thus, as I've indicated to you, in this case, the term negligence is meant to be—to be defined or is defined, really, as the failure of the Red Cross to use the care, skill, and learning ordinarily possessed and used by blood collectors in the same or similar circumstances."

Then, after telling the jury that the standard of care was "defined as . . . the skill and learning ordinarily possessed and used by blood collectors," Salzman issued a conflicting instruction: the care ordinarily possessed and used did not set the standard of care.

Roland Ray's attorneys expected the jury to be utterly confused. Feldman hoped that when the jury returned with questions, the definition could be righted.

Still, jury confusion prior to closing was dangerous. "We knew this had the potential for real disaster," Mike Feldman would later recall.

In his closing statements, Feldman sought to drive home the meaning of standard of care—what was "reasonable and prudent, not what was ordinarily done."

Feldman told the jury, "Fifty seconds. Fifty seconds. One moment in time. That is all it would have taken to have prevented this tragedy. One moment with a donor. One moment of caring as much about the person receiving the blood as they cared about the person giving the blood. One moment of caring as much about people as politics. That is all it would have taken."

The jury's decision was important, Feldman explained to them, "There may be blood bankers sitting in boardrooms across the country waiting to hear the outcome of this case." But its verdict was more important to Roland and Janet Ray. "They want to see an injustice corrected. Roland and Janet Ray want the Red Cross to stand up and acknowledge their mistakes. And they haven't done it. We ask that you let them know that they made mistakes."

After reiterating the various points made by expert witnesses and the document exhibits, Feldman concluded.

"Roland Ray is a good, hardworking and decent man with three children that he loves and a wife that he loves, but his life will never be the same, since he received that letter and the emotional pain that went with it. I would like to tell you, don't feel that pain. But you have to think about it. You have to remember it because it's the only way you can do your job. It's the only way you can evaluate the damages. Your verdict will, in a very real way, put a value on Roland Ray's life. And I'm very sorry to say, that your verdict is the only way to give meaning to Roland Ray's death.

After a short recess, Peter Bleakley began his closing remarks on behalf of the Red Cross. He chronicled the Red Cross's role in implementing the National Blood Policy, which eliminated paid donors who "weren't as safe" as volunteer donors. Creating the resulting volunteer system had been a daunting task, but one which, he explained, the Red Cross undertook to "save lives [and] make the blood supply as safe as reasonably possible." The Red Cross did "its very best" in the face of hepatitis in the 1970s and the disease known as AIDS in the early 1980s. "But blood was not safe one hundred percent then, it wasn't safe one hundred percent before hepatitis, and it isn't safe today. It is a human organism. There has been no way established on the record of this case to make blood one hundred percent safe." And that, he said, "was an unfortunate fact."

"It was just not the obligation of the Red Cross to make blood one hundred percent safe," Bleakley told the jury. "The obligation of the American Red Cross, which is accepted and accepts, was to make the blood supply as safe as reasonably possible."

Red Cross found that its existing screening methods were "effective, as effective as you could prove them to be until a test was available."

Bleakley then said the evidence in this case concluded that "direct questioning was not the way to go and that the form of screening procedures employed by the Red Cross, namely, self-deferral, the use of a combination of this pamphlet and the donor card, was the standard of care."

And the standard of care was all blood bankers had to abide by. "Did the standard of care in existence in July 1984 require the asking of the direct questions as to donor's sexual high-risks?" That, Bleakley said, was the issue before the jury.

After a brief rebuttal by Mike Feldman, the jury went into deliberation. Feldman was feeling upbeat. He believed he and Chris and Peter had tried a good case. If the somber manner of the Red Cross counsel waiting in the hall was any indication, the jury was going to find in Roland Ray's favor.

A day and a half later, predictably confused, the foreman sent a note to the judge: "How do prevailing practices affect the finding of the standard of care? Please explain."

This was the chance Feldman had been awaiting. He told the judge, "Given the fact that the only question that they have asked us about had to do with prevailing practices, and since counsel for both sides were in agreement that the best way to clarify the conflict is by reading only the prevailing practice instruction—"

The judge cut him off. He decided to give both the standard of care definition and the prevailing practice instruction.

After another day of deliberation, the jury queried the judge again. It could not resolve whether the Red Cross had complied with the standard. Feldman again requested that Salzman clarify the issue by reading only the prevailing practice instruction. Salzman cut him short. "Counsel, the court has made a decision. I've done that."

It was then that Feldman thought the case was dead for Roland Ray. He walked into the hall feeling sick to his stomach. If the standard of care was defined as prevailing practices—doing what everyone else was doing—then he didn't have a shot in hell proving the Red Cross negligent. He saw that the attorneys for the Red Cross were now smiling and laughing.

During the course of nearly three years, Mike Feldman had come to know and admire his client. His initial impression of this blue-eyed, six-foot-four gentle giant, so different from him in background and temperament, had been confirmed. Roland Ray was an extraordinary man.

Feldman felt heartsick at what might be awaiting him.

On the second day of jury deliberation, Roland was listening to the soft cadence of the voices of his wife, his mother, and his sister as they sat with him in the hallway. For them, talking passed the time. He had once been a lot more garrulous. That was before the shooting. Since then he had become quieter, a more pensive man.

Still, the women's voices were comforting, and in their predictable rhythm, Roland let his mind wander. His life had become something unfamiliar to him. He had been traveling uncharted territory, he had had to turn within for guidance. Mike Feldman had told him to be prepared for what could be a negative verdict. Roland refused to believe him.

He felt sure the jury would find on his behalf. So when they returned to the courtroom on the afternoon of May 20, his stomach was in knots. Then it happened fast.

The court asked the foreman: "Do you find that the Red Cross's efforts to screen out blood at high-risk of AIDS in July 1984 met the standard of care required of a reasonable and product blood banker at that time?"

The foreman said, "Yes."

Mike Feldman jumped to his feet. He was already thinking about the appeal. "Your Honor," he said, "I would like permission to talk with the jury."

The jury was under no obligation to discuss the case with counsel, but it agreed and permission was granted. Feldman wanted to know their thought process. How did the conflicting definitions of standard of care influence their decision? By the time he left the jury room, Feldman was convinced that had the court's instruction been clear, Roland Ray's faith in the people would have been borne out.

Roland sat alone in the empty courtroom. He had told his wife and mother and sister to go back home and he would follow. The bottom had fallen out of his stomach and he simply did not have the ability to stand up and walk out. His thoughts turned back to that night years earlier. He had made all kinds of bargains with God. Today, waiting for the verdict, he had done the same. Before, he had been praying for life. This time, he had been praying for justice.

Your donor tested positive for the virus associated with AIDS. There was no way to know the donor was infected.

When he had received that letter, five years after the transfusion, he had called the Red Cross in Washington D.C.. He told the woman at the switchboard what had happened, that he wasn't looking to place blame, only for some answers. She connected him to yet another woman, who sounded very nervous. He was told to call the AIDS Hotline.

It was as if they were just trying to get rid of him.

He told Janet what had happened. How can you destroy someone's entire life and just turn your back?

If you are well, then you probably have not been exposed.

He was well.

Now, in the courtroom, Roland heard the whir of sirens from the streets below.

Hey, Magic Man!

There was no magic to make this right.

CHAPTER SIXTEEN

ALBATROSS

1994

The [regional] boards have been used to deceive the American public, the legal system, our local communities, local unions, and our employees when it was convenient for the American Red Cross. That's the kind of albatross the regions have around their necks.

Dr. William Swallow
Former Red Cross Regional Board Chairman

In the months following the Consent Decree for federal injunction, Red Cross executive vice president of Blood Services Fred Kyle had managed to wrest his division from the control of Mrs. Dole's Special Team. While her political handlers were polishing their boss's tarnished image, Kyle got down to the operational streamlining he had previously attempted. As a result, by the fall of 1993, there had finally been advances in addressing safety and communications issues. The fifty testing labs had been consolidated into ten. The number of computer systems had been reduced and the goal of a single state-of-the-art system was becoming more feasible.

But Fred Kyle had long since recognized that to Mrs. Dole, form was more important than substance. Progress notwithstanding, he knew he was as vulnerable as his predecessor, Dr. Jeff McCullough, had been. McCullough, Kyle learned, had experienced the kind of second-guessing that continually usurped the very expertise for which he was hired.

On a trip to Portland, Oregon, Kyle discussed his concerns with a former Red Cross Board member, Buzz Braley. Braley had served as an elected member of the National Board of Governors from 1986 to 1992 and as chairman of the volunteer Biomedical Services Committee, the oversight board for Biomedical Services. An auto dealer,

Braley had an affiliation with the Red Cross that dated back to the late 1970s, when he had been chairman of the Portland region. Having committed himself to learning about blood banking, Buzz Braley considered himself well versed in service operations.

Braley knew that Mrs. Dole had lured Kyle from a lucrative position at SmithKline, and that he had made a substantial sacrifice in pay and lifestyle. "The carrot that drew Fred Kyle," Braley recalled, "was doing something wonderful for the Red Cross. He was a superb choice."

Over lunch, Braley listened as Kyle recounted his distress at the discrepancy between the Red Cross's public image and its operational practices. He told of who was in who was out, who was supposed to shoulder the blame for the 1993 injunction. How he had been instructed to fire certain regional officials who, in his judgment, were simply convenient scapegoats. And how he had to "run through a gauntlet to get Mrs. Dole's attention."

Braley knew what Kyle meant. He, too, had raised questions about the influence of Mrs. Dole's Special Team, particularly her longtime loyalist Jenna Dorn and retired General William Reno, who headed up national operations. "Everybody was subject to their 'view,' shall we say," Braley explained. "I believe they really didn't have the depth of knowledge of biomedical services. They didn't seem to understand what it really was about. They were terribly concerned about the perception of the Red Cross outside, publicly, PR-wise."

On his return from the West Coast, Fred Kyle was called into the office of Elizabeth Dole. Subsequently, he tendered his resignation, effective December 1993. A high-level Red Cross official privy to what had transpired at that meeting said, "Kyle told her, 'Look, I'm not here to support your political program. I'm leaving.' "

Karen Shoos Lipton, Red Cross's forty-one-year-old general counsel, was slotted into Kyle's position in an interim measure.

"What hurt the Red Cross," Braley explained, "is that Mrs. Dole has been able to attract very talented people, but they come and go. She'd get some real winner and then something happens, maybe they're not brought into the team, and they don't stay, especially in Biomedical Services."

The consulting firm chosen to conduct the second internal review was BDM International Inc., one of the clients of Michael Goldfarb's Washington, D.C. consulting firm. Until 1988, one of the largest publicly held defense contractors in the world, BDM was hired not only to evaluate Blood Services but to advise ways to fix what it found was wrong. BDM's consulting tab amounted to $3.68 million for fiscal 1994.

Pivotal to this newest overhaul was a change in the Red Cross's culture from social service model to that of a large corporate entity operating in an intensely regulated environment. In a letter to board chairman Norm Augustine, Mrs. Dole emphasized that a more business-like structure "will make Blood Services consistent with a corporate model of a regulated entity operating under a single license."

The "sweeping national reorganization" of Blood Services was announced by Elizabeth Dole on April 15, 1994. Several new positions were created at headquarters, including vice presidents for regulatory affairs, information systems, and strategic planning. Those officials would report directly to a new senior vice president, the chief executive officer for blood operations. In order to establish what Mrs. Dole termed a "smaller and smarter" headquarters, a temporary "modified freeze" on new hiring and budget action was put into effect in all regions. Local blood boards would be stripped of their long-held personnel and budget responsibilities. The intent was to structure and run each center uniformly so that FDA's regulatory expectations and requirements could be met. There would be "increased resource sharing among regions."

The Red Cross was also making efforts to centralize quality assurance training. It had, a month earlier, announced the establishment of a national biomedical services "training college" in Fairfax County, Virginia, so that, Mrs. Dole explained, "the patches and pins worn by Red Crossers will serve as emblems of excellence in the industry."

By tightening control at headquarters, the Red Cross intended to establish and monitor one set of standards and practices to ensure "one unassailable level of quality and safety."

"When I announced Transformation three years ago," Mrs. Dole told the press, "I promised we would no longer continue to patch and bandage a system that evolved in the early 1940s. . . . We are leaving behind the last vestiges of our old system, one in which our Red Cross culture of local autonomy was not consistent with achieving a unified, state-of-the-art blood system."

She also announced the resignation of then head of Blood Services Dr. Peter Tomasulo. Like Kyle, the soft-spoken Tomasulo had joined the Red Cross with a sense of mission. He, too, left profoundly disillusioned. Within months, general counsel Karen Shoos Lipton would also quit, after having served over a decade with the Red Cross. Bright and well respected, Lipton was, like Kyle and Tomasulo, reportedly distressed by the increasing authority of the Special Team.

Commenting on Lipton's resignation to become CEO of the American Association of Blood Banks, Dr. William Swallow observed, "Someone of her caliber looking at the high turnover in senior management and deciding to go to AABB tells me she saw the writing on the wall as far as management was concerned at the Red Cross." Other high-level officials pointed to the control exerted by the Special Team as prompting the departure of highly qualified personnel. One former official at headquarters explained, "In all objectivity, I don't think the Special Team enhanced anything. They hindered things. I wish they'd have left us alone."

The Red Cross had a mighty task ahead, if the FDA inspection reports for 1994 were any indication. A year after federal imposition of more stringent standards and severe repercussions should the Red Cross fail to comply, violations nationwide in the acquisition, testing, manufacturing, and distribution of blood persisted. As a result, blood which tested reactive for HIV, hepatitis, syphilis, and other infectious agents had been released, and hundreds of units of blood and blood products were recalled.

According to the Lewiston, Idaho *Morning Tribune,* over a 4-year period, 18,000 units of blood had been recalled from the Lewis and Clark region in Boise. FDA inspections cited Boise for lack of cleanliness, inadequate quality control, and malfunctioning equipment. Donor files and blood processing procedures were deficient. FDA had documented similar violations at Boise in 1990, 1991, and 1992. FDA enforcement reports in 1994 indicate that 300 units which tested HIV reactive, or were simply not tested, were released to Montana, New Jersey, Florida, Michigan, California, New York, and the Netherlands.

On February 23, 1994, the FDA warned Red Cross headquarters of the failure of its Lewis and Clark region to comply fully with the Consent Decree. "This letter is to provide you notice that unless you demonstrate or achieve compliance with the applicable standards and regulations, it is the intent of the FDA to institute proceedings to revoke U.S. License 0190-011. Additionally, pursuant to the criteria for notification outlined in paragraph VI.A of the May 12, 1993, Consent Decree of Permanent Injunction, the FDA is herein notifying the ARC of the agency's determination that the ARC has failed to fully comply with the Consent Decree, failed to follow ARC standard operating procedures (SOP), and violated the law." Boise was ordered to submit to FDA within ten days a written plan offering specific action to effect compliance with all applicable regulations and standards and specific time frames for such action.

The Red Cross responded by shutting down its Lewis and Clark blood region, including two blood banks in Montana. It planned to reopen the facility in three weeks, when a new management team was recruited; and employees were retrained, an independent quality assurance team was assembled, and hundreds of operating procedures were assessed by a team of experts. The center would, in fact, not be up and running until August. Blood testing was transferred to St. Paul or Detroit.

FDA did not go so far as to threaten license revocation at the Peoria, Illinois blood center, but it did demand immediate corrective action. During inspections between April 25 and June 3, 1994, the FDA cited multiple violations, including the failure to maintain accurate records to identify suitable donors and track the final destination of blood products. The inspection reports also showed that in 1993, the Peoria facility lost track of a dozen units of blood or blood products, released more than 1,000 units of outdated red blood cells, and shipped 144 units of blood products to out-of-state hospitals without a federal license. Computer glitches mistakenly identified as eligible several permanently deferred donors, including one who was a high risk for HIV and another who had tested positive for hepatitis B. No efforts were made to rectify discrepancies and duplications in donor files.

Despite Mrs. Dole's center-by-center Transformation, inadequately trained collection staff and volunteers in Peoria were responsible for nearly 300 errors in 1993 and 1994. The result: over 60 ineligible donors were accepted, deferral codes were wrongly recorded 50 times, incomplete medical histories of donors were taken, collection bags were mislabeled, and instrumentation was not properly maintained to assure proper function. Doses delivered by the blood irradiator had not been checked for 4 years.

On December 29, 1994, FDA wrote to Brian McDonough, chief operating officer of the Red Cross Blood Services, "FDA investigators documented numerous deviations from FDA law, regulations, and the requirements of the May 12, 1993 Consent Decree of Permanent Injunction."

On January 11, 1995, the Red Cross responded, citing numerous steps taken by the heart of America region to correct deficiencies.

The FDA's 1994 inspections documented similar operational transgressions in Nashville. Nashville had taken three years to notify 14 donors of their HIV-reactive blood test results, and it had closed Look-Back cases before the disposition of HIV-reactive blood and frozen plasma had been determined. The center also lost track of 2,003 units of blood and blood products, more than two dozen of which showed positive viral markers or had been marked for deferrals. No attempt was made by blood bank personnel to determine where the missing units had been sent.

Glitches in Nashville's computer system altered donor codes and identification numbers and deleted donors from the deferral lists. At least five donations had been accepted from an unsuitable donor. FDA also cited the facility for shipping 267 units out of state without a license.

FDA cited the Miami Red Cross for having lost over 3,000 units of blood and blood components, 197 of which had tested reactive for viruses or had been rejected as unsuitable. In addition, 18 pints of blood were released in a two-month period from blood donors for whom Red Cross had taken incomplete medical histories. Despite these violations, Miami continued to operate uninterrupted. "If public health had been at risk," headquarters insisted, "we would have moved to shut it down."

In Rochester, 175 units of HIV-reactive blood were released between 1985 and 1994 from three dozen donors who first tested HIV reactive in 1985 but were not entered into the donor deferral registry. Those donors gave blood 28 times, some as recently as May 1994. Blood from 16 other donors who had tested reactive for HIV between July 1992 and June 1993 was also released for processing. System errors prevented the recall of HIV-reactive blood donated prior to 1991. Since products like frozen plasma have a 10-year shelf life, there was no way to identify contaminated products donated before 1991, which were still on the market.

In Savannah, Georgia, a pheresis donor whose platelets had tested reactive for HIV in 1993 was allowed to donate twice in 1994. Units of red cells were shipped from the center without any indication that

HIV testing had been performed. In Lansing, Michigan and Cleveland, Ohio, donors with a history of cancer were allowed to give blood repeatedly, despite federal regulations requiring their disqualification.

Federally mandated HIV Look-Back programs were not properly carried out in Rochester, Atlanta, Georgia, Columbia, Charlotte, and Birmingham. A Mobile donor who tested reactive for HIV in 1993 had since donated blood under three different names. His file had been closed prior to identifying all his aliases and before tracking his 1993 donations. In Huntington, West Virginia, components manufactured from the blood of an HIV-reactive donor had not been tracked. The donor had been implicated in 4 cases of transfusion AIDS; he had already died. The center failed to track other products made from other HIV-reactive donors and took up to five years to open several investigations into suspected transfusion AIDS cases dating from 1988 and 1990. Huntington further failed to investigate suspected cases of post-transfusion hepatitis involving 44 donors.

Recalls of tainted product were conducted throughout the system. FDA reports listed hundreds of Red Cross blood products recalled under two categories: Class II, defined as "a situation in which use or exposure to a volatile product may cause temporary or medically reversible health consequences or where probability of serious adverse health consequences is remote," and Class III, "a situation in which use or exposure to a volatile product is not likely to cause adverse health effects." Over a dozen Red Cross centers released blood that was potentially tainted with HIV, hepatitis, staphylococcus, streptococcus, and other bacteria and viruses onto the market. The other reasons for the recalls ranged from errors in testing to mistakes in recording donor eligibility to mislabeling of blood products.

Some of the largest recalls occurred in Syracuse, New York and Lansing, Michigan, where it was discovered in May 1994 that technicians had been misreading syphilis test results for a year. The error in interpreting test results had been noted five months before a recall was issued. Faulty syphilis testing also resulted in the recall of 2,000 units released by Baltimore and 210 units released by Dedham, Massachusetts. An FDA inspector wrote that since donors who test positive for syphilis were considered to be at high risk for AIDS, failure to properly interpret the syphilis tests meant "donors who should have been deferred due to an AIDS-related risk cannot be identified."

Most devastating was the Red Cross and Miles, Inc. recall of tens of millions of dollars worth of plasma derivatives from a donor who died of Creutzfeldt-Jakob Disease. CJD is a rare degenerative neurological disorder thought to be caused by a virus-like agent. The donor had given fifty times. The financial repercussions of this recall would be felt well into 1995.

Baxter Travenol issued a worldwide recall of its immune globulin intravenous product when patients in Spain and Sweden contracted hepatitis C. Baxter manufactured the same product, Gamaguard, for the Red Cross under the name Polygam, which it also recalled "just to be absolutely on the safe side."

In Philadelphia, unidentified errors in hepatitis tests resulted in 142 improperly tested units released. Lost blood plagued the Midwest, South, and East. Springfield, Missouri mislaid 1,568 units. Wichita lost 331 outdated units, Mobile six units, and Birmingham 10 units, including a unit from an HIV-reactive donor. Baltimore lost track of 270 products in a two-year period. After several costly false starts, the long-promised single computer system to provide more reliable data on blood safety still had not been installed. Mrs. Dole had extended her time frame to at least another two years.

While potentially contaminated blood continued to plague its supply, the Red Cross vigorously opposed the Blood Safety Act of 1994. The legislation required doctors to advise patients before elective surgery about the option of autologous self-donation as a guarantee against AIDS, hepatitis, and other blood-borne diseases. The act also required doctors to discuss directed donations from relatives. Although the Red Cross acknowledged that self-donation was safest, it argued that blood from relatives could be even more dangerous than the blood of a stranger. Relatives would lie, the Red Cross claimed, about the risk factors. The Blood Safety Act passed the Senate but was killed in House.

The Senate unanimously approved an amendment that made it a federal crime for persons who tested positive for HIV and had received "actual notice of that fact" to "knowingly donate" or "attempt to donate" blood. The amendment's sponsor, Senator Jesse Helms of North Carolina, pointed out, "If carjacking is a federal crime, and Congress has voted to make it so, Congress should do the same for those irresponsibly mean-spirited people who knowingly donate infected blood and other bodily fluids." The bill authorized criminal penalties of up to ten years in prison and a $20,000 fine.

That same summer, Jimmy Ross, a retired four-star general who directed Army logistics for the Persian Gulf War, was selected by Mrs. Dole to head Red Cross Blood Services. He had been recommended by former Secretary of Defense Dick Cheney and former chairman of the Joint Chief of Staffs General Colin Powell. Brian McDonough, former head of the Red Cross in St. Louis, remained as chief operating officer for Blood Services.

Meanwhile, on the regional level, rebellion stirred within the ranks of the Red Cross's volunteer boards. Wilkes-Barre's Dr. Bill Swallow, had intuitively sensed headquarters' skewed motives years earlier. But it was not until the annual Red Cross convention in Seattle in the summer of 1994 that he received more tangible confirmation. "Mrs. Dole was there," he recalled, "for the fluff, for the opening remarks, the rah-rah that went on. As far as the nitty-gritty, nuts-and-bolts breaking the news to the regional people, she stayed away from that." The news was this: regional boards, long the backbone of Red Cross volunteerism, would be divested of their responsibilities for financial and personnel decision making. The regions would no longer be the employer of record: headquarters would assume that function, in essence nationalizing all employees. Volunteers, headquarters had decided, had little place in this new set-up.

The rationale behind this move, which went to the core of Red Cross's local social service culture, was, management told attendees, the FDA Consent Decree. Red Cross had decided to take absolute control based on FDA's regulatory requirements.

Representatives of the regional boards were outraged. For nearly ninety years the local board of each area had developed and run largely autonomous local organizations with little input from National Headquarters. The tradition of the Red Cross not only had given the impression of local self-containment, but it was a de facto recognition by National Headquarters itself that each board had such powers. As a result, blood regions had been able to secure necessary local funding, volunteers, and donors.

Swallow was stunned at the announcement. On what basis did National presume control down to each and every employee, when it did not even know how many local employees it had or what their needs were? Where had the Consent Decree stated, or even implied, that such control was required for regulatory compliance? What headquarters was implying was that regional board mismanagement was cause of its financial and regulatory woes.

Swallow would later recall, "It was a power thing. It smelled bad."

So great was the outcry at the Seattle annual convention that Hap LeVander, chairman of the Biomedical Services Committee, convened a committee. The intent was to rewrite more relevant roles and responsibilities for regional boards. Management at headquarters assured the committee that its recommendations would be seriously considered. Heading that committee was Pat Powers, a board chair from the Ohio region. Swallow was a member.

Their first meeting on June 14 reflected the regions' frustration. Members agreed that there was no conceivable way Washington, D.C. could deal with local employees on an adequate and equitable basis. Local community ownership of regions and participation of volunteers were critical. If you took away that sense of community, it wouldn't be long before the donors would just stop coming.

It seemed to Swallow that National needed and had found, a scapegoat for its own "inept management." The plasma recall fell right at the feet of headquarters, for one. The FDA had taken issue with the way Red Cross's Holland Labs was conducting confirmatory HIV tests. Blood which tested positive for the HIV antibody at the regions was sent to the D.C. lab, where the more specific Western Blot test was conducted. The FDA challenged the accuracy of Holland's test procedures. As a result of safety questions, about $42 million in albumin, a plasma-related product, had to be quarantined by June. That stymied necessary cash flow at a time when headquarters was fast approaching crisis. Its $150 million debt overload was fast approaching.

The way Swallow saw it, "Headquarters didn't give a damn about the volunteers. All headquarters wants the volunteers to do is stick out their arm and provide them with a free resource, and they, in turn, process and sell it at a profit in order to continue to feed the coffers of Washington."

As the summer wore on, the committee seemed to Swallow to grow more acquiescent to headquarters' initial proposition. The more vocally opposed became more compliant. As a result, the Powers committee recommendations were "watered down." Swallow felt compelled to make known that the resulting recommendations did not reflect the consensus. In an August 18 letter to Richard McFerson, chairman of the Biomedical Services Committee, Swallow expressed his distress at the "many disheartening situations with respect to the problems that National Headquarters has had and continues to have with respect to management," particularly in regard to Transformation. "Three and one half years and 150 million dollars later, American Red Cross Blood Services has virtually nothing to show for the time and expense. We now have a consent decree that will more than likely be in force for years. We have an unstable senior management structure, we have a national laboratory that has been shut down because of faulty testing, we have tens of millions of dollars of product quarantined due to faulty testing. The money taken from the pension fund to drive this Transformation has only succeeded in creating tremendous distrust between the regional staff and national management. What do you think that the American public would conclude if they were aware of these situations?" Swallow asked. "How long do you think the American Red Cross Blood Services can function under the proposed changes when the American public is made aware of the rationale truly behind this restructuring?"

He asked McFerson to allow a representative group of chairpersons to present a minority report to the Biomedical Services Committee.

In an August 31 letter, McFerson responded that Swallow's request was poorly timed. He would, he wrote, attempt to arrange a meeting in which Swallow could discuss his concerns with Norm Augustine, Elizabeth Dole, and other appropriate individuals. McFerson's letter arrived on September 6, one day before the committee was scheduled to meet. A subsequent letter from McFerson indicated that the Biomedical Services board had voted unanimously to approve the Powers committee recommendation. Swallow wrote back that his dissenting opinion was shared by a "closely knit network of regional chairs." He again requested a meeting with Elizabeth Dole and senior management; there was no response from McFerson. The recommendations of the Powers committee would not be implemented. Nor would they, as management had assured, be integrated into the bylaws. The entire exercise appeared to be a way to let volunteers blow off steam.

As the year wore on, the financial picture at headquarters looked bleak. Blood Services revenues had dropped over $1 million from 1993. Expenses increased over $50 million. Red Cross's deficiency of revenues over expense and property acquisition was a high $57 million, compared to $5.6 million the prior year. In 1993 assets were $200 million; in 1994, $143 million. In October, headquarters called for an across-the-board financial clampdown of the regions. In an October 7 memo, Jimmy Ross and Blood Services COO Brian McDonough informed senior principal officers of the money crunch resulting from the plasma quarantine. The market value of the withheld plasma-derived products was approaching $90 million. Consequently, plasma products were generating a "negative cash flow" compared to projected budgeted cash inflows of about $4 million per month. It would be, Ross and McDonough told the regional heads, "many months before the cash flows from plasma products are fully restored."

The quarantine coincided with heavy outlays for Transformation. To finance Transformation investments and compensate for operating deficits from plasma, Biomedical Services at headquarters had to seek about $50 million from external funding sources. To minimize that borrowing, headquarters had deferred credits to the regions for fresh-frozen plasma sent for fractionation. Those credits had been used by regions to pay off their debts to National arising from purchases of necessary goods and services and the long required per [blood] unit assessments, a sort of "fee" imposed on regions by headquarters. National was now asking for cash settlements on accounts. Headquarters was assessing regional finance needs. It would determine whether those needs could be met by cash transfers from other, more prosperous regions.

Swallow had Wilkes-Barre's accountant work up some scenarios based on headquarters' dictates. The worst case put the region out of business in forty-five days; the best, ten months. "They'd have killed us," Swallow recalled. Wilkes-Barre refused to acknowledge the new no-credit system and would not pay National. It also refused to loan interregionally.

A follow-up memo dated October 25 from Jimmy Ross and Brian McDonough reported that Biomedical Services had imposed yet more controls on the regions. Those "special measures" to conserve cash, limit external borrowing, and cut costs included a controlled hiring freeze, freezing of capital expenditures except for essential regulated equipment, and deferral of purchase of vehicles in order to cut the equipment budget, which was about $8 million. Only essential travel was permitted, in hopes of eliminating about 20 percent of that yearly $15 million budget. Interest charges on sector loans would remain in effect and regions were expected to continue to settle their liabilities with headquarters.

The financial squeeze hit some of the most prosperous regions hardest. There were massive layoffs. No merit raises were given. Employees had to pay for their benefits packages. Distrust festered. In Louisville, Kentucky, director Dr. David Jenkins felt headquarters had tied his hands. The morale problem had become so severe that his staff had contacted the Teamsters to intercede on their behalf. Jenkins was able to negotiate an eleventh-hour agreement, but the schism left its mark. "People felt very alienated, underpaid. They had lost faith," he said.

The Teamsters did have to intervene on behalf of Red Cross workers in the Greater Chesapeake–Potomac region, which served Maryland, Washington, northern Virginia, and South Central Pennsylvania. Wages had been frozen for all 800 employees to offset regional losses of $832,000 in the first quarter of 1994. To lure donors and boost blood product sales, the region was employing tactics which raised eyebrows among some of its blood banking peers. The center offered cash bonuses—as high as $600 each quarter—to recruiters who successfully solicited blood donations. It offered medical clients significant blood discounts. One marketing ploy was dubbed by the *Philadelphia Inquirer* the "blue platelet special." Luxury cars were perks for top managers. Inside sources at C&P spoke of "dying baby" sob stories concocted by motivated recruiters to fill quotas.

Regional layoffs and wage and hiring freezes notwithstanding, many officials at headquarters remained cushioned by six-figure salaries, and, as often, six-figure expense accounts. Jenna Dorn was earning over $161,000. Peter Page, now senior principal officer for the North Atlantic region, pulled in $231,000. Richard LeGrand, senior principal officer for the Western region, was paid nearly $200,000, plus $118,310 for expenses and other allowances. Vice president of business development Geoffrey Deutsch received a $178,841 paycheck, plus over $86,000 for expenses. Stephen Stachelski, Jr., the new vice president of quality assurance (a system which still had not been fully implemented) was paid $241,000, plus nearly $24,000 for expenses. Another 131 employees at headquarters earned in excess of $50,000; the Red Cross's 1994 tax return did not indicate just how much in excess.

Consultants were still cornering the big money payouts. Special Team member Michael Goldfarb earned over $300,000 in one year from the Red Cross. For fiscal 1994, J. Walter Thompson Advertising was paid over $4 million, this apart from media time donated to the Red Cross. BDM International followed as the second highest paid consultant, at $3,686,317, and West Coast Direct Response direct mail earned $1.79 million.

In an attempt to attract contributors, headquarters was reassessing its fundraising pitch. John Thomas, senior vice president for development, told the *Chronicle of Philanthropy* in early 1994, "We tend to treat solicitations as a kind of drive-by shooting where we gun them down, solicit them, and go on to the next donor. That's not the way we can do business anymore."

Despite money woes, strikes, and regional board schisms, Elizabeth Dole managed to endure. Women Executives in State Government honored her with their Lifetime Achievement Award. She was selected for induction into the Safety and Health Hall of Fame I nternational for what her press department described as "her numerous transportation, workplace, and blood safety accomplishments." She accepted the Radcliffe College Medal and even created a new award category at the North Carolina Press Association, receiving its first "North Carolina of the Year" distinction. She was identified by a Gallup poll has one of the world's ten most admired women. Only a month after the FDA's order for permanent injunction was put into effect, Red Cross's president was presented with the 1993 Norman Vincent Peale Award for Positive Thinking. She told a rapt audience at the Plaza Hotel in New York City, "My plate is full, and there is still so much to be done. The important thing for me is to constantly seek God's will and try to follow His plan."

In a year-end interview with the *New York Times*, Special Team member Mari Maseng-Will said of Mrs. Dole, "She's always been a woman of a lot of power and force . . . a strong and effective woman [who] did not threaten people and could still be a leader."

CHAPTER SEVENTEEN

TWO CHILDREN

Anthony brings music to our ears.
Often we let go of a tear.

Kimberly Ann Cochran, age 15
Anthony Kirby's cousin

Steve Choquette had been skeptical the Red Cross would force the Anthony Kirby case, known as *Jason Doe v. American National Red Cross*, to trial. Anthony's young life had been hideous since 1988. Connie and Darrell were rock-solid parents, active in the PTA and in local charities. Connie herself had been a two-gallon donor to the Red Cross. It seemed to the Holland & Hart attorney that the blood bank would prefer to settle this one.

By the spring of 1993, the implicated surgeon and anesthesiologist had reached an out-of-court settlement with the Kirbys. The physicians had, however, stayed in the suit long enough to give their consent for the Red Cross to remove the case to federal court. There, the Red Cross had failed to win its argument that as a governmental agency it was immune from jury trials and punitive damages. U.S. District Judge Charles Haden had ruled that while the Red Cross engaged in government work, it did not have federal immunity from lawsuits. He also ruled that Congress chartered the Red Cross as a "private commercial enterprise," not as a public agency. Haden was the first judge to explain the Red Cross's lack of immunity in a detailed written opinion. His ruling went against other decisions rendered in favor of the Red Cross in numerous courts.

To win punitive damages, the Kirbys would have to prove that the

Red Cross and the Charleston Area Medical Center had acted in a "willful, wanton, reckless, or malicious manner." Choquette and Sonny Flowers, intended to show that given the information available about AIDS in 1983, Anthony's life could have been spared through precautionary measures, including surrogate testing and direct donor questioning. Lawyers for the defense would claim that the blood bank and hospital did take proper precautions against HIV contamination. Jurors would have to decide whether the Red Cross should have followed the advice of the Centers for Disease Control, which suggested tough screening of gay and drug-using donors, or the organization's own "Joint Statement," which advocated self-deferral.

Specifically, the jury would be asked, based on the standard practices in effect in the blood banking profession in August 1983, was the defendant, the American National Red Cross, negligent? Were practices established by the blood banking profession as a whole negligent in August 1983? And, judging the Red Cross's conduct against blood banking practices that *should* have been in effect in August 1983, was it negligent? Last, did the Red Cross's negligence proximately cause Anthony Kirby's infection with the AIDS virus?

Since June, Holland & Hart had been battling Arnold & Porter for every square inch of territory, from document production to admission of evidence. Choquette, Flowers and their West Virginia co-counsel had to resort, in virtually every instance, to court intervention compelling the Red Cross to comply. The Red Cross did comply, while lodging lengthy formal objections at nearly every turn. It was particularly resistant on the blood donor issue and refused to disclose the donor's identity. The Kirbys' lawyers had managed, however, to reconstruct sufficient documentation to determine who the donor had been. An honorably discharged military veteran with an exemplary employment record, the thirty-nine-year-old man whose blood Anthony Kirby had received had donated regularly every sixty days for three years at the Red Cross Center in Huntington, West Virginia. The Red Cross was ordered to confirm the identity of the already deceased donor, who had told a physician, upon his being diagnosed with HIV that he was a homosexual and that he and his partner had been monogamous save for an "occasional escapde." Moreover, he had tested core antibody reactive. Look-Back records left no doubt that this donor had infected more than one person.

By January 1994, settlement negotiations in the Kirby case fell apart and the trial date was set for April in Charleston, West Virginia.

The Red Cross had two potential advantages. At the time of Anthony's surgery, the Red Cross argued it had had limited knowledge of transfusion AIDS. Strategically, the donor's death could also work in its favor. The organization could decide to lay the blame for negligence on the donor.

A "command central" was set up at Holland & Hart, where roughly a dozen attorneys were simultaneously working on about nine other transfusion AIDS lawsuits. Of the five against the Red Cross, two besides the Kirby case involved children. In one, a young woman in Tennessee had infected her baby following surgery; both died within an eighteen-month period. In Oklahoma, an infant had been transfused with HIV-infected blood in the spring of 1984. The child was still alive and nearing her teens. The remaining three cases charged United Blood Services, a non–Red Cross blood bank, with negligence.

In 1994, the Red Cross tallied up some major victories and suffered some setbacks in federal courts nationwide.

Significantly, its litigation strategy was supported by a U.S. Court of Appeals decision holding that a 1992 Supreme Court decision authorizing Red Cross to remove cases from state to federal court applied to all cases filed against Red Cross, both before *and* after that decision. Within thirty days after that ruling, Red Cross lawyers in Philadelphia alone removed more than two dozen suits pending in state court to federal court. The Red Cross was also successfully claiming protection under state blood shield laws, statutes of limitations restricting the filing of malpractice claims, and its quasi-governmental status, which it argued, insulated it from jury trials and punitive damages. The most reliable argument remained the standard of care issue.

However, its statute of limitations argument proved ineffective in California, where an appellate court decided that the time limit had not expired in the case of a thirteen-year-old who had acquired AIDS by transfusion with Red Cross blood when he was four.

Holland & Hart also successfully challenged the Red Cross's claim to immunity as a quasi-governmental agency in U.S. District Court in Wisconsin. *Jane Doe v. American National Red Cross* was pursued by the wife of a surgery patient who had died of transfusion AIDS. The HIV-tainted blood had come from the Red Cross's St. Paul blood center. The court rejected the Red Cross's argument that its status as a federal "instrumentality" precluded it from facing trial by jury, but it did rule that the Red Cross could not be held liable for punitive damages. The court reasoned that the governmental services the Red Cross provided under its charter—specifically, military support and disaster relief—could be jeopardized by a large punitive award. In September, the Red Cross would settle the $7.5 million suit for an undisclosed amount.

The Red Cross also did not fare well in two cases in Pennsylvania which had far-reaching legal implications for the organization. In one case it settled with the transfusion-AIDS patient, but its codefendant, the Osteopathic Medical Center of Philadelphia, successfully petitioned the court to compel the Red Cross to remain in the case through trial and verdict. The U.S. Court of Appeals in Pennsylvania also heard arguments in the case of victim Carol Marcella, who had been infected during a 1985 emergency transfusion. In 1995, it would reject the Red Cross's claim that as an "agency" of the federal government, it was protected from jury trial. The court ruled, "The Red Cross is not given wholesale governmental immunity simply by virtue of its federal charter." Marcella was allowed to pursue donor discovery and deposition, as long as the donor's identity was kept confidential. The court found that donors' rights to privacy "must be balanced against victims' needs to establish their claims and against the state's interest in preserving the integrity of the volunteer blood donor system." The donor, a homosexual male, had tested HIV positive after a second donation.

An earlier non-Red Cross decision in New Jersey which was later upheld had significant implications for the Red Cross. A Bergen County jury ordered the American Association of Blood Banks to pay $405,000 to a Fairlawn heart surgery patient who had contracted transfusion AIDS in 1984. AABB was found negligent for failing to require member blood banks to implement surrogate testing and for not aggressively questioning the donor's sexual history. David Schrager, a Philadelphia attorney, founder of the AIDS Litigation Group of the Association of Trial Lawyers of America, termed the decision an "important verdict because it imposes liability on a trade association which has presumed to set suggested standards for the industry." The verdict was one of the early cracks in the blood industry's long-standing previously effective "standards of care" defense.

Compounding its legal defeats, the Red Cross's plasma recalls that year placed its lucrative Baxter Travenol relationship in a disquieting spotlight. Baxter was among four manufacturers of antihemophiliac factor named in an unprecedented class action lawsuit.

The suit was brought in September 1993 in the federal courthouse in Chicago on behalf of about 9,000 persons with hemophilia who were infected with HIV and their infected partners, children, and/or survivors. In a chilling affirmation of Dr. Donald Francis's 1982 predictions, the *Common Factor,* a newsletter published by the Committee of Ten Thousand, who had brought the lawsuit, wrote twelve years later, "Like the canaries in the coal mine, persons with hemophilia serve as the early warning system for the nation's blood supply. We all contracted hepatitis B, then non A-non B hepatitis (hepatitis C), and then HIV. The hemophilia community has provided gravesful of information about the safety of the blood supply."

Rhone-Poulenc Rorer, the parent corporation of Armour Pharmaceutical; Miles/Cutter, Baxter Healthcare Corporation, owners of Hyland Therapeutics, which processed Red Cross plasma; and Alpha Therapeutics, owned by Japanese Green Cross were charged with pursuing aggressive advertising and marketing strategies to sell AHF products, while downplaying the significant risks of viral infection and AIDS. By July 1982, the suit alleged, the drug companies knew their product was contaminated with AIDS, yet they chose not to warn users. The National Hemophiliac Foundation, which was also a defendant, continued to promote factor concentrate. Withdrawal of the product at that time would have required pulling approximately $100 million in AHF concentrate off the market, significantly reducing corporate profits until newer, safer product became available.

Half of the country's 20,000 hemophiliacs and 80 percent of those with severe cases had been infected with HIV through clotting factor used in the early 1980s. By 1993, sixty percent of the total U.S. hemophiliac population had died.

A team of ten law firms prosecuting the claim was expected to petition the federal court to make available thousands of documents, including drug company memos and government papers. The National Hemophilia Foundation was opposing the class certification, the final step necessary for the families to proceed to trial.

The Washington D.C. Red Cross had decided to take to trial only one transfusion-AIDS case represented by Ashcraft & Gerel: that of Roland Ray. The case was on appeal, based on misdirection of the jury on the part of the court. The Red Cross had settled Ashcraft & Gerel's other cases, including the Michaels triplet case. Only days before the Kirby trial, Hailey Michaels had died of AIDS. She had not survived to her tenth birthday.

That same month, ten-year-old Anthony Kirby had taken a turn for the worse. In January, Connie Kirby and her husband had withdrawn him from classes in favor of home schooling, principally to avert his catching flus and colds. Anthony attended occasional high school basketball meets as an observer and sometimes stopped by school during lunch breaks to visit his friends. Connie had told the mothers of his closest friends about his being HIV positive, and there was little interruption of his afterschool play dates. Earlier, there had been a few parents who'd attempted to cause trouble at school. They had petitioned to prevent Anthony—still known anonymously as the "HIV-infected child"—from playing sports and participating in other activities. But that furor had died down, largely due to the school principal's efforts to hold AIDS education meetings for the public.

The little boy was stoic about his poor health and told his mother he did not want to talk about his illness. He was receiving nutrients from his "happy meal," as well as a variety of antibiotics and morphine to relieve the pain in his limbs. He would, though, protest taking baths and oral medication. "Wait a minute!" he'd say. That was Connie's sign that her son wasn't yet ready to swallow the pills or get into the bathwater, which, he said, hurt his skin. Anthony had so little control over his life that "Wait a minute!" gave him a measure of empowerment.

Harris Teeter, a corporate sponsor of the Charlotte Hornets, had learned about Anthony's AIDS and his love of basketball. In early spring, the sponsor presented the Kirby family with four front-row tickets. The morning of the Hornets game, Anthony was running a high fever, but he wept so bitterly at the prospect of staying home that his mother acquiesced. She packed his "barf bucket," filled his "happy meal," and made sure he had sufficient morphine. For most of the game, Anthony stood, eating nachos and cheese and cheering. A friend bought him a Hornets jacket and a cap. A week later, Anthony was barely able to walk. He was quickly debilitated by recurring fevers, diarrhea, and early-stage pneumonia. The morphine doses were increased.

The Kirbys had planned to attend the trial and testify. Connie now told Steve Choquette her place was with her son. She was caring for Anthony eighteen hours a day and supervising several shifts of nurses.

Darrell made the trip to West Virginia for the trial and each night reported back to Connie what had transpired that day. Days before the trial, Steve Choquette had developed walking pneumonia and would spend a portion of his time in the emergency room of St. Francis Hospital. He would handle some of the questioning at trial, but Holland & Hart partner, Bruce Jones took over much of the case. Jones shared the burden with Sonny Flowers and the Kirbys' local lawyers, Joe Caldwell, a tenacious Vietnam vet, and his partner, Chuck Riffee.

The Jason Doe (Anthony Kirby) case opened with a significant impairment. During discovery, Holland & Hart discovered further negligence on the part of the Red Cross and the Charleston Area Medical Center. The issue concerned the Red Cross Look-Back. The blood bank had known in mid-1988 that HIV-infected blood had been sent to CAMC in 1983. It did not notify CAMC of that fact until January 1990 by regular first class mail. The hospital claimed it did not receive the letter and therefore did not take any steps to notify the Kirbys. It was only through Dr. Frank Saulsbury's diligence that CAMC acknowledged its receipt of the bad blood. "For nineteen months, the Red Cross sat on that information and didn't so much as convey it to the hospital," Choquette later recalled. "Getting the word out should have been a four-alarm fire for the hospital and the blood bank, but they didn't even send up a smoke alarm." To him, this was a clear-cut instance of wanton negligence.

Choquette and his colleagues attempted to amend the initial complaint to include this improper handling of Look-Back. The Red Cross and CAMC argued that they had not had adequate opportunity to prepare a defense on this point. The judge denied Choquette's request to allow the Look-Back issue at trial.

Nevertheless, on the eve of the trial, CAMC decided to settle for an undisclosed amount, leaving the Red Cross the sole defendant.

The Kirby team's prediction that the Red Cross would attribute negligence to the deceased donor was borne out by Peter Bleakley's opening remarks. Prefacing his comments with references to the industry's lack of knowledge of blood-borne AIDS in 1983 and its apparent restriction to "fast-lane" gays, the Arnold & Porter attorney went on to describe the Red Cross's on-site donor education. The donor had been handed a pamphlet and told to sit down and read it, as well as the insert about AIDS high-risk groups. He was asked to sign a document stating that he had understood the pamphlet. He answered a health history questionnaire and he filled out a donor card that referenced symptoms of hepatitis and IV drug use. Then he was sent to a cubicle, where he was asked by an intake nurse whether he'd read and understood the pamphlet.

True, Bleakley acknowledged, no direct questions about sexual behavior had been asked, but that had not been required by either the industry or the FDA. Still, the donor had had adequate information to make the decision to defer from giving blood.

Many of the witnesses on behalf of the Kirbys were familiar faces on the transfusion AIDS circuit, among them Dr. Don Francis, Dr. Marcus Conant, and Dr. Frank Saulsbury. Their testimony attempted to demonstrate that the Red Cross had not taken adequate precautions to protect its blood supply from HIV in 1983 and had failed to meet federal guidelines for donor interviews. In anticipation of the Red Cross's attempt to blame the donor, the Kirbys' attorneys had a communications professor testify as an expert witness. Lawrence Ray Wheeless, of the University of Texas, a former faculty member at West Virginia University and Marshall University, told the court that the leaflet's language was cold, bureaucratic, and impersonal. Wheeless said it was poorly crafted and difficult to understand, and its references to high-risk donors vague. The intent of the information was diluted by extensive peppering of the words "giving," "good neighbor," and "as long as we work together."

When it came time for Frank Saulsbury to discuss Anthony's prognosis, Steve Choquette suggested that Darrell Kirby leave the room. Kirby declined. He remained in the courtroom as the University of Virginia physician related to a slack-jawed jury the boy's deterioration. "Most children with AIDS die a slow and painful and difficult death," Saulsbury testified. "I don't expect him to be any different. His mother and father have gone above and beyond the call of parents. It's hard for any parent to throw in the towel, to drop back and stop. It's going to be hard for them to back off."

Another of Anthony's physicians, Dr. Penelope Muelenaer, testified that when the child entered the hospital's intensive care unit, "a number of people thought he wouldn't come out." She almost broke down when she described Anthony's struggles and his progression to the point of being allowed to make an outing to a videogame arcade with hospital staff. "Caring for a child like this was difficult for all of us," Dr. Muelenaer said. "How well he's done is a tribute to his parents' devotion. His mother's positive attitude encouraged all of us."

By April 12, Anthony showed improvement and the Kirbys' local physician, Dr. Ron Overstreet, approved the trip to West Virginia. Connie placed her son under the care of her mother, who lived in Charleston. While unpacking her bags, she found a neatly folded piece of paper. It read, "My mom is special to me. She helps me take a bath and she buys me food. My mom takes me places like the grocery store and out to eat. She helps me do my medicine. She loves me very much, and I love her, too."

Connie had thought she had cried all her tears, until she saw that letter.

She had been apprehensive about testifying, fearing a replay of what had occurred the prior year. In February 1993 she had submitted to two days of depositions conducted by the defendants' counsel. She had been asked every conceivable personal question, from her weight to whether she had had sex with anyone other than her husband. Connie understood that Arnold & Porter had a job to do, but was that kind of humiliation necessary? Steve Choquette and Bruce Jones had counseled her to restrain her emotion in court. She promised herself she would. Connie held up well during her twenty-minute testimony, even when she described the trip to Toys "Я" Us to buy Anthony rollerblades. "He looked at the rollerblades and then he became agitated and he said, 'Mom, get me out of here. I want to go home.' It was the first time he had realized his limitations." Anthony knew then that he would not roller-skate or ride his bike again.

It was only when Connie stood up from the witness box and walked down the aisle toward the door that she cried.

Among the Red Cross's first witnesses was a former CDC medical officer. Dr. Jim Allen had since left government and was a top executive with the American Medical Association. Allen countered the testimony of Don Francis. He testified that in 1983, AIDS investigators had just begun to narrow their search for the causal factors and explore possible links to sexually active homosexual men and that little was then known.

One of the Red Cross's more effective witnesses was Dr. Mabel Stevenson, former Blood Services director for the Red Cross Tri State region in Huntington, West Virginia. Stevenson testified she had followed Public Health Service guidelines. "Based on the information I had, I believed our blood supply was as safe as it possibly could be," Stevenson told the court. The same month Anthony contracted the virus through Huntington's tainted blood, Stevenson called a press conference to solicit more donations. She had told the media, "We rely on our donors' truthfulness about their medical history. We can't take any precautions we aren't already taking." AIDS was not a threat, according to the Red Cross's reckoning then.

Equally effective was the intake nurse at the blood center. Rickie Ann Sizemore testified that she would never have asked donors about their sexual habits had the setting not been confidential. The donor had, she said, every opportunity to say that he was gay and had had multiple partners. Dr. Gerald Sandler, associate director of Red Cross Blood Services in the 1980s, told the jury that he had worked with health groups to learn the source of AIDS transmission, and that early cases were not linked to blood transfusion. Theories about transmission were numerous, but no one source had been yet pinpointed. And there was a concern, Sandler said, about discouraging donors. "People don't come flocking to the centers," he told the court. Subsequently, Red Cross witness Dr. Amoz Chernoff, former head of the Division of Blood Diseases and Blood Resources for the National Institutes of Health, testified that NIH's studies had not favored surrogate testing. But, Chernoff conceded that the federal bureaucracy was ponderously slow.

Prior to closing remarks, the Red Cross moved for a directed verdict on punitive damages. Arnold & Porter claimed that evidence against the Red Cross did not demonstrate "wanton, willful, or grossly negligent conduct," that would allow the jury to decide on punitive damages, since the Kirbys' attorneys had anticipated the Red Cross's motion. They had not been permitted to introduce the linchpin of their punitive damage case: the Look-Back evidence. That evidence, which was ruled inadmissible, showed the kind of negligence and wanton disregard for human life which Choquette believed, would have given the jury "the full picture to go all the way. They would have found not only negligence, but causation."

But the jury would not learn of the improper Look-Back.

Haden removed the punitive damages issue but he ruled that the jury could still determine whether the Red Cross should compensate the child and his parents for their pain and suffering, as well as for the financial burden of Anthony's illness; those costs approached $500,000.

In his closing remarks, Bruce Jones told the court, "The Red Cross took a risk that AIDS was a one-in-a-million risk, that it wasn't the tip of an iceberg, that it would stay in New York and San Francisco. When the Red Cross took that gamble, they were playing with the lives of helpless people like that infant in the hospital in this state." Peter Bleakley closed his defense citing data that indicated AIDS was seemingly confined to a cluster of big cities. "The data did not provide those same results would be found across the United States in medium-sized cities and in West Virginia," he explained. "In 1983 there were more questions than answers, and science doesn't jump to conclusions."

Several days into their deliberation, the jury requested transcripts of testimony from the plaintiff's witnesses. The Red Cross opposed that request, but the judge allowed the transcripts. Later that day, the jury told Haden that they might be headed for a deadlock. No unanimous decision had been reached. In a note to the judge, the foreperson wrote, "we don't see an end in sight." Haden encouraged them to proceed. He canceled his own plans to attend a federal case management seminar so that he could answer their questions. The jury again requested transcripts.

The next day, April 26, the jury returned. After three full days of deliberating, the members prefaced their verdict with a request to the judge. They told Haden they did not wish to discuss the case with either counsel and asked for an escort by court marshals to their cars. Haden called the court to order, and each of the four questions originally posed to the jury was asked. Had the Red Cross been negligent based on the standard practices in effect in August 1983? The jury answered, "No."

Had practices established by the blood banking profession as a whole been negligent in August 1983?

The jury answered, "Yes."

The Kirbys' attorneys were stunned. This sweeping indictment of the industry had followed an essential absolution of the Red Cross's culpability.

As to question number three: judging the Red Cross's conduct against industry practice that *should* have been in effect during that time, was the Red Cross negligent? The jury answered, "Yes."

But the jury found that Red Cross's negligence did not cause Jason Doe's (Anthony Kirby) infection with AIDS. Years later, that decision would still baffle Choquette and his colleagues. Nonetheless, the case represented the first time the Red Cross and the blood banking industry had been found negligent at trial.

Following the verdict, the Red Cross decided to settle each of Holland & Hart's pending cases in one fell swoop. The Kirby case had been, Choquette explained, too close a call. "I think they recognized we had gotten favorable legal rulings, more than anyone in the country. They weighed the odds and what we had accomplished and concluded it was in their economic and legal best interest to settle."

On June 1, 1994, Dr. Frank Saulsbury sent a somber letter to the Kirby family physician, Ron Overstreet. The University of Virginia specialist had examined Anthony on May 31, the boy's eleventh birthday. The usual laboratory tests were conducted, as well as a chest X ray. Saulsbury wrote, "I spent considerable time discussing Anthony's recent deterioration with his mother. I think she is aware that he has slipped considerably over the past few months and that his outlook in the relatively near future is quite dismal. Mrs. Kirby is comfortable with our current approach of empiric therapy and a nonaggressive approach to diagnostic studies. I think that she will be amenable to withdrawal of some of the drugs when the time comes. At this time, however, I can't think of any drugs that we can discontinue without having a major adverse effect on his remaining life. Obviously, there will come a time when we will want to provide only comfort measures. I think his mother is aware of this eventuality."

Saulsbury had run out of any "bright ideas at this juncture." Antibiotics might diminish the boy's fevers and pulmonary symptoms. "I wish I had something more to add, but I think we are getting close to the end of the line here and I am not sure that anything we do is going to have a major influence at this time."

Outside one of the windows of Anthony's downstairs bedroom, he could see the swing set his parents had bought for his fifth birthday. It had been years since he had played on those swings. He no longer had the energy even to feed his goldfish, Mo, Larry, and Curly. Beside the aquarium, Anthony had hung a large photo of a rainforest frog. On the opposite wall was a photo of a red Lamborghini car. His baseball bat and glove and his two favorite hats, a Mickey Mouse hat and the Hornets cap, hung on the wall beside his bed. When his older brother came home from his part-time summer job, they would play Uno card games. Mathew would read aloud Anthony's books about animals or the rainforests. Sometimes Anthony would just say, "Hold me, Mathew," and Matt would take him in his arms and quietly look out the window at the trees and creek.

Connie had told her husband that she would know when it was time for Anthony to go. She now believed the time was approaching. She believed Anthony knew, too. On a trip to Chuck E Cheese for his birthday, he brought with him hundreds of arcade game coupons he had been saving. This trip, he spent every single one, buying little prizes for his family and nurses. He had none left.

On the evening of June 21, Anthony lay listless. Now and then his face contorted with pain. Connie and Darrell sat beside him. In a small voice, he told his parents he was tired of being sick. Connie asked him if he wanted to be with Jesus. Anthony said, "Yes."

She told him it was all right, that if he wanted to go, then it was all right for him to go.

From midnight to about four in the morning, Anthony lay half sleeping, saying nothing. Connie, Darrell, his favorite aunt, Margaret, and his cousin Diane were beside him. Mat came downstairs for a while, but the sight of his brother in pain, looking like a little old man, scared him. The night was dark and quiet. There was only the muffled sound of the creek through the open window and the soft drone of the refrigerator that held Anthony's medicines.

Shortly after four A.M., Anthony suddenly said in a clear, strong voice, "Wait a minute!" Connie jumped. Several minutes later, Anthony again called out, "I said, 'Wait a minute!' " This time he was more adamant.

Then he was gone.

They buried him on June 26, in the family plot at Sunset Memorial Gardens in Charleston. They dressed him in his Hornets jacket and cap, teal soccer shorts, and a white T-shirt. The granite marker was engraved with a baseball hat, mitt, and ball. Connie had placed in her son's casket his Davis Edmond doll. The doll's once bald head was covered with bandaids.

That evening, alone in her mother's living room, Connie closed her eyes and dozed off. She was awakened by a very light kiss on her cheek. There was no one in the room. "It was my son," Connie would later recall thinking. "It was Anthony saying, 'I'm okay.' "

CHAPTER EIGHTEEN

MANIFEST DESTINY

1995

Red Cross used a national disaster to perpetuate a fraud on the public.

Dr. Ron Gilcher
Oklahoma Blood Institute

At 9:02 A.M. on April 19, 1995, a nearby explosion wracked the Oklahoma Blood Institute at the corner of Tenth and Lincoln in Oklahoma City. The two-story brick building seemed to sway on its foundation, then set itself right. Framed pictures fell off the walls; glass shattered. Dr. Ron Gilcher, OBI's CEO, felt the blast at his home fourteen miles away. It sounded to him like a plane had crashed. Tinker Air Force Base was close by and Gilcher phoned into his office, expecting confirmation of an accident. He was told, instead, that a building downtown had blown up. What caused the blast, and the extent of the damage and injuries were as yet unknown.

An oncologist and hematologist who had headed up OBI since its founding in 1977, Gilcher was recovering from an illness that had almost left him paralyzed. But within minutes of speaking with his secretary, he was in his car, barreling down Interstate 40, following the path of spiraling, sooty clouds. Smoke clouds meant burn victims and the need for blood. From home, Gilcher had already dispatched reserves to Oklahoma City's hospitals, principally the "universal donor," Type O. Type O could be received in an emergency by any patient, regardless of blood type.

It had been fourteen years since the city had been hit by a major disaster. In 1981, a boiler had exploded in one of the grade schools, killing several children and injuring many. Hundreds of people had turned out to give blood at the community blood bank, which served the needs of all Oklahoma City hospitals and most in Central Oklahoma. There were usually between 2,000 and 2,500 units of blood on OBI's shelves. Whatever this latest crisis, Gilcher knew he could expect highly motivated support. Oklahoma City was that kind of community, tight knit, accessible. It was on this communal spirit that OBI had built an international reputation and a reliable donor base of 400,000 in a town of 950,000.

As Dr. Gilcher drove to OBI, Dr. Ron Gillum, chief of clinical pathology at the University of Oklahoma College of Medicine, was checking blood supplies at the hospital's Transfusion Services. Media reports had placed the blast, a bomb explosion, at the Alfred P. Murrah Federal Building at NW Sixth and Robinson. Gillum knew bombs meant more deaths than injuries, the need to match body parts to ID victims when only a limb was found. The hospital could expect glass shard wounds, which might require surgery if fragments were lodged in or near arteries. The gas tanks of cars parked near the Murrah Building had apparently caught fire, which accounted for the dark smoke. Transfusion Services assured him it was well stocked by OBI in case of burn trauma. Gillum dispatched medical school faculty and residents to the two other clinical labs he supervised—Children's Hospital and the Veterans Hospital. He also sent several pathology residents to OBI to screen donors and free up blood bank staff for other critical work.

At 10 A.M. Ron Gilcher cleared the police barricades and pulled up to the blood center. More than 200 donors were already lined up outside OBI, which was only one-sixth of a mile from the Murrah Building. Donors would be coming in at a rate of 300 to 400 an hour. By the end of that first day, 4,200 people would give blood at OBI; a total of 9,000 would donate within the next three days. OBI's fixed donation sites in the metro areas were, by midmorning, reporting overwhelming support, a tripling, even quadrupling of numbers. Nearly 700 community residents waited to give blood at the American Fidelity Bank. Deer Creek High School logged in 560 donors. At Tinker's 72nd Air Base Wing, several hundred personnel were processed as donors. The Clarion Hotel, which had been hosting a banquet, sent the luncheon food on to OBI and became a donor site. The city's fast food vendors also delivered, unsolicited and unpaid, quantities of pizza and sandwiches to the blood bank, which had begun to resemble a military command post.

There were friends, neighbors, and relatives in the Murrah Building. Gilcher would learn that forty-seven of the victims had been OBI donors. OBI's Drive Coordinator at IRS, Edye Smith, would become the human face of the disaster. Her sons, Chase, age three, and Colton, age two, died in the building's daycare center.

Dr. Don Rhinehart, OBI's chairman, had just completed his first surgery at St. Anthony's Hospital when the blast hit. Rhinehart was the hospital's chair of the Division of Neurosurgery and a cofounder of OBI. Shortly after the blast a messenger arrived at St. Anthony's with a box containing 25 units of blood from Red Cross in Tulsa, over 100 miles away. Most of the victims were being sent to St. Anthony, which was only blocks from the Murrah Building, but its blood supply from OBI was more than adequate. The receiving staff did not know what to do with this Red Cross blood. The only Red Cross presence in Oklahoma City was a disaster services chapter. Tulsa had had minimal contact with Oklahoma City hospitals—a few secondary contracts for specialty orders of blood. But Tulsa often had trouble filling those occasional orders. Unlike OBI, it had a donor recruitment problem.

Rhinehart sent the messenger to the Department of Pathology. But pathology had not placed any order. The surgeon then phoned Ron Gilcher and asked what was going on.

A TV had been set up in the secretarial area of OBI to keep track of developments. Any available radios were also tuned to the news. Within hours, Elizabeth Dole was on-site for a CNN interview. When asked "What's the status of the blood supply," Mrs. Dole replied, "Well, the most important thing that people can do is to call this number, 1-800-HELP NOW, and offer financial resources. If they can give money, then we can obtain whatever might be necessary. That's the most effective way to help now."

Mrs. Dole's open-ended response served Red Cross blood centers in Wichita Falls, Kansas; Waco, Texas; St. Louis, Missouri; and Little Rock, Arkansas, which launched immediate blood drives, specifically, they announced, for the bombing victims. Tulsa and its satellite center in Norman, twenty-five miles from Oklahoma City, were also aggressively appealing for blood for the victims. By the afternoon of April 19, Tulsa Red Cross had issued two urgent press releases; the first cited "numerous calls" from donors and the need for blood, "for surgeries that may be scheduled for victims of the explosions." The second release, entitled Red Cross Responds Immediately to Help Oklahoma City Explosion Victims, described Red

Cross involvement: "Responding to news of the tragic Oklahoma City explosion this morning, blood donors from around the Southwest Region streamed into Red Cross collection centers as they opened in Tulsa, Norman, Waco, and Wichita Falls. As a result, the anticipated need has been fully met. About 3,000 volunteers regionwide turned out to give blood, resulting in almost 1,000 units actually collected from determined donors."

But this release qualified its appeal. The Red Cross indicated that it had contacted the Oklahoma Blood Institute and that "there is no immediate need for extra blood donations. However, we never know when the next disaster might strike. The Red Cross encourages people to donate any time throughout the year."

Tulsa Red Cross spokesperson Melissa Kozicki told the *Norman Transcript*, "This [bombing] is causing a tremendous drain on our blood supply. We provide blood to the metro area and will need all blood types." Kozicki later claimed she was misquoted not only by the Norman press but by all state media, who ran her appeal.

As for blood donation ads, she speculated, "Maybe they were placed by well-meaning people using the Red Cross."

The Cleveland Chapter of the Red Cross was also soliciting blood donors, who would be "desperately needed in the days and weeks to come due to the bombing in Oklahoma City." The Red Cross in Woodward, Oklahoma told the public that donors would "probably" be needed "the rest of the week." On April 20, the Red Cross's national headquarters issued its own statement thanking "Americans across the country offering help in the aftermath of the Oklahoma disaster." As to offers of blood, "While your blood donations will most probably not be needed for the victims of the Oklahoma City disaster, they will be essential to saving lives throughout the critical summer months."

Well into May, the Red Cross was placing blood donation ads and sponsoring community blood drives to, as its mid-Central Oklahoma chapter put it, "help the victims of the April 19 bombing." A year later, the organization ran a full-page ad in the Blackwell, Oklahoma *Journal-Tribune* for a bloodmobile drive. The attention grabber, which featured a drawing of an angel ("Be an Angel, Give the Gift of Life"), told readers, "One year ago on April 19, a devastating disaster struck at the heart of our state in Oklahoma City. Almost immediately, processed blood given by the Red Cross donors at community drives in our area was en route to Oklahoma City to fill that critical need. You may not be able to be a Red Cross disaster volunteer. You can be a Red Cross blood donor!"

But no Red Cross blood was requested or used by Oklahoma City hospitals treating the bombing victims on April 19 or at any later date. The sole box of blood which had been sent from the Tulsa Red Cross to St. Anthony had been sent back. OBI had met all the blood needs caused by the disaster.

But the bombing disaster profited the Southwestern region of Red Cross. On an average day that region drew approximately 500 donated units; Tulsa approximately 250 units. On April 19, 1995, the region drew 1,000 units from about 3,000 donors—within hours. At an average price of between $55 to $75 per unit, that blood drive stocked the region's depleted shelves, and the coffers of a deficit-plagued system—under the banner of aiding the Oklahoma City victims.

In June, Gilcher wrote an angry letter to Red Cross vice president of communications Roy Clason. He conveyed his distress at the Red Cross's misuse of a national disaster to build its donor and client base. The organization's misrepresentations were undermining Oklahoma at a time when unity was essential. Gilcher told Clason that the Red Cross's implication that the emergency blood needs had been met by its own donors was "not true." In fact, Red Cross had not even offered OBI the kind of assistance local blood banks had. "When a disaster/crisis requiring blood support occurs in the United States, the ethical and professional methods of handling that need has been and should continue to be that neighboring blood centers (Red Cross and non–Red Cross) should call the primary blood center and offer support if it is needed," Gilcher wrote. "The Oklahoma Blood Institute received many calls from non–Red Cross centers offering help. No call was made by the Tulsa Red Cross to offer help to OBI. Instead, the Tulsa Red Cross acted in an unprofessional and unethical manner at the time of the Oklahoma City explosion."

In the wake of the bombing, Tulsa had also been intruding on OBI's donor pool. It had contacted every large OBI donor group in the Oklahoma City area, asking that they conduct additional blood drives with the Red Cross. "This behavior has left a very unfavorable impression of the American Red Cross with many of our donor groups," Gilcher told Clason. "We would not like to see this negative reaction mistakenly transferred to the Oklahoma County Chapter of the American Red Cross, with whom we work closely. Not only has this been confusing, a waste of time, and unpleasant for donor groups, but it has cost our recruitment staff a great deal of production time in responding to many calls from upset blood drive coordinators."

The Red Cross was, Gilcher learned, also trying to gain a foothold in Oklahoma City's hospitals by undercutting OBI's already low prices.

On July 5, Jimmy Ross, senior vice president of Biomedical Services at Red Cross National Headquarters, responded to Gilcher's letter to Clason: "As to your charges that the Red Cross took advantage of the bombing tragedy, I was dismayed by them. Nothing could be further from the truth. Our actions reflect nothing more than the Red Cross's readiness in responding to a public disaster of unknown proportions, even in the early hours, when the goal of 'emergency relief' organizations—including hospitals, ambulances, and blood centers in and out of the state—is to be prepared for the worst."

To Gilcher, quite another message was being conveyed to the public, one of "clear cut deception, fraud." He explained, "American Red Cross believes they are infallible, that they can do anything, get away with anything. They don't believe they are accountable to the people."

As far as the University of Oklahoma's College of Medicine pathologist Ron Gillum was concerned, "The Republican presidential candidate's wife will have to be held accountable as to what's going on."

While Red Cross was seeking to expand its territories, its own blood regions were plagued by employee unrest, dissatisfied clients, deficits, and in many cases persistent federal violations of blood safety laws. In March, 134 unionized blood collection workers at the Red Cross in Atlanta went on strike. Employees were angered by pay cuts and longer hours. The strike ended after 37 days, when headquarters agreed to certain demands. In July, approximately 100 Detroit Red Cross workers went on strike. The Red Cross blood centers in Joplin, Missouri, and Springdale, Arkansas shut down as a result of dispute for local control. But nowhere were the repercussions of discontent resonating more than in the Greater Ozarks, where, by August, 100 Red Cross employees had walked out of the Springfield, Missouri center to start up their own community blood bank.

When Don Thomson went to work for the Red Cross in Springfield as its administrator, the blood center had $37,000 in cash and securities, a failed capital fund campaign, and was barely meeting the blood product needs of local hospitals. That was in 1988. Three years later, as Springfield's principal officer, Thomson and a highly motivated staff and community turned around the blood bank. Within five years, it had paid back a community loan of half a million dollars, was more than meeting hospital requirements, and had built a cash reserve of $1.8 million.

A retired Air Force pilot and Defense Department procurement officer, Thomson initially viewed blood banking as just another precision manufacturing operation. He did not expect his job to become his passion. "I'd spent years supporting activities that would kill or maim people," he explained. "Now, I was seeing this miracle taking place, saving people's lives." Thomson was also witnessing massive changes stemming from Transformation. The resulting consolidations were straining the financial and manpower resources of the Red Cross blood centers nationwide. Arbitrary decisions coming down from headquarters failed to account for local needs. In March 1995, headquarters ordered Thomson to raise fees to his customers by six percent, charge ten percent more for certain blood types, and charge at least ten percent more to hospitals who were not exclusive to the Red Cross. Following a lawsuit brought by Lifesource, a community blood bank in St. Louis, the Red Cross rethought its pricing for nonexclusive clients.

For several months in 1994, Thomson had been assigned temporarily to assist in St. Louis's recovery from an FDA crackdown on violations. St. Louis had been run by Brian McDonough, who had been promoted to chief operating officer at headquarters. The center was, Thomson recalled, "an absolute mess." About forty percent of certain blood products were not meeting quality standards, he said. The blood bank had lost millions of dollars. Pricing was so haphazard that hospital buyers referred to fees as the "deal of the day." The acrimony was palpable. Thomson returned to Springfield to find as discouraged an environment. Headquarters had ordered more than half of Springfield's financial reserves sent to cash-strapped St. Louis and Little Rock, Arkansas. Thomson was also told to start drawing more blood. "They were asking us to bleed more, and pay more."

As he saw it, the essential grassroots, reciprocal nature of blood banking had been supplanted by institutional arrogance. Thomson and three board members quit.

Throughout that summer many more Springfield Red Cross personnel resigned, each for his own reasons. For public relations manager Gene Waite, a minister who had been with the Red Cross for twenty-one years, it was the organization's shift from a humanitarian effort, to a corporate commodity brokering. For others it was an unacceptable pay and benefits scale that placed the Ozarks at a disadvantage. For one well-respected officer, a comment made by a medical official at headquarters sent her packing. When she asked whether Springfield would ever see a return on its money from its blood exports, she was told, "The sooner you get this through your head, the happier you'll be. It was never your money."

Other Springfield personnel worried about the instability at headquarters, its lack of engagement with the community. There were rumors of layoff and personnel relocation.

For most, the final straw was the noncompete agreement. On June 16, Thomson and several board members had flown to D.C. to meet with Brian McDonough. They hoped to arrange an amicable agreement to buy out the Red Cross center in Springfield and convert it back to a community blood bank. Headquarters refused their offer. Undeterred, on June 19, Thomson and colleagues filed articles of incorporation to establish the Community Blood Center of the Ozarks. Their operational models were Dr. Bill Swallow's Wilkes-Barre, Pennsylvania blood bank and the Louisville center run by Dr. David Jenkins.

Several regional hospitals, which were dissatisfied with the Red Cross product quality and the absence of local community control, lent the fledging blood center $3 million dollars to start up. The Community Blood Center of Greater Kansas City temporarily included it under its FDA license and gave it technical support. A site was found. Community leaders helped negotiate favorable financing. Donor groups at colleges, city utilities, and manufacturing plants throughout southeast Missouri and northeast Arkansas opened their doors to the new center's blood drives. A local board of directors was appointed with responsibility for hiring all staff.

By mid-July, six officers who had resigned from the Springfield Red Cross center has joined the CBC.

The Red Cross moved fast. It attempted but failed to seek protection under a Missouri state law concerning competetive blood banking activities to prevent CBC from entering the blood business. In July, headquarters presented its remaining local staff a "nondisclosure/noncompete" agreement. In exchange for a "lump sum monetary payment" of between $1,000 and $2,500 and "continued employment in the region," signees would have to "abide by reasonable limits on the types of employment they may seek within the area served by the region." Since the Red Cross employee relationship was legally "at-will," the organization had the right to impose certain employment conditions and to change them as it deemed appropriate. Rejection of those terms, as indicated by a refusal to sign the agreement, "would be treated as having given notice of resignation." Employees would thus forfeit not only severance pay, but benefits accrued by longtime service to the Red Cross. The intent of the agreement was, the Red Cross claimed, "to protect ARCBS's (American Red Cross Blood Services) legitimate interests in keeping its trade secrets and proprietary information confidential and to prevent competitors from gaining an unfair advantage by using the knowledge, expertise, and relationships of the Red Cross, largely or exclusively at the expense of ARCBS."

Only four managers signed. By late August, 100 of the 176 Red Cross employees—many of whom had been with the organization for more than 20 years—resigned. Among them: two thirds of the nursing staff, most of the donor recruiters, and the maintenance crew. Some had been at the threshold of receiving retirement benefits. It didn't matter to them. The sense of betrayal was profound. Resignation had become a matter of conscience.

Springfield's two major hospitals, St. John's and Cox Medical Center, signed supplier agreements with CBC. By the fall, eighty-three percent of the Red Cross's hospital clients had turned to the community blood bank for their product.

On December 21, the Red Cross sued CBC. It charged the principals with "tortious interference with a business expectancy, misappropriation of trade secrets, and tampering with computer data." The complaint contended that CBC had induced the Red Cross employees to leave, raided the Red Cross files, and interfered with the Red Cross's relationship with its blood donors. The Red Cross was also seeking a temporary restraining order against the blood bank. After a telephone hearing the following day, the court denied the Red Cross's request to enjoin CBC from exploiting its "trade secrets." It also denied the Red Cross's request to order the return by CBC of certain allegedly confidential, misappropriated materials. But the court consigned to enjoin CBC and others from destroying any such materials and records.

When the court heard the case on January 17, 1996, it would find "virtually all of the evidence presented by the Red Cross was successfully refuted or otherwise explained away by CBC's witnesses." The Red Cross's evidence was deemed "insufficient" and the court denied its request for a restraining order. The judge did issue a scathing indictment of this battle over blood. He criticized CBC for "intransigent" behavior, which stoked the combative "rapacious" struggle. As for the Red Cross's action, "Plaintiff has only itself to blame for its present predicament. Its arrogance in insisting that its national vision be imposed upon Southwest Missouri, whether or not it fit, was the first act of aggression. Its ill-advised it's my way or the highway approach failed to account for the fierce independence of the residents of Southwest Missouri. A concession here. . . . a mere willingness to listen and bend would likely have avoided the morass in which it now finds itself."

The Red Cross subsequently amended its lawsuit to include the four major hospitals which had signed with CBC.

The Red Cross's actions in Oklahoma City and Springfield reflected a corporate strategy of expansionism aimed at positioning the organization as the nation's principal, if not sole, blood provider. Its 1995 internal documents revealed a highly competitive, aggressive strategy for nationalization, one which factored in economic variables such as market share and competition. One of those documents, the business plan for the coming years, defined the Red Cross goals succinctly: "The organization's strategic intent [is] to become the preeminent nationwide provider of blood, plasma, and tissue services. . . . Other than defending market share, ARCBS will expand into new markets in an effort to increase revenues and drive down fully allocated per unit costs." Noting its own high costs in an already price-sensitive arena, "ARCBS [American Red Cross Blood Services] could easily trigger a price war which they are financially unequipped to fight. Thus the expansion must be very selective and creatively pursued in order to minimize market disruption."

There was a wall map hanging in the Rosslyn, Virginia office of Chief Operating Officer Brian McDonough. Areas serviced by Red Cross blood banks were marked in red. "White areas," as they were referred to internally, were regions serviced by community blood banks and thus targets for the Red Cross development.

The documents further noted that headquarters had made several market assumptions. First, "a drop in blood collections industrywide favors ARCBS, keeping demand (fees) high and maximizing the value of the unique advantages ARCBS has in collections, including name recognition and respect, its volunteer support, and its national economies of scale." Secondly, "commoditization of blood components and the downward pressure on prices ultimately favors the largest player who should be able to achieve unique economies of scale, making it more difficult for competitors to fight a gorilla [sic] war in discreet niches." While there was an "increasing willingness of blood centers to compete," ARCBS could "leverage its size in negotiating favorable access" to technologies and products, "amortize their costs over much larger volume and roll them out quickly through a centrally managed system." Furthermore, the changing nature of healthcare delivery, which "favors strategic alliances, will influence ARCBS marketing/distributing strategies."

The Red Cross identified blood as a commodity rather than a service. In fact, hospitals considering developing their own blood banks were pegged as Red Cross "competitors" in the fight for market share in blood. As the business plan indicated, "The primary competitor to the Red Cross will be the hospitals themselves. It is anticipated that hospital associations, in which a group of hospitals agree to consolidate their laboratories and blood banks into one, or at least fewer, shared operations, will offer stiff competition."

In an attempt to head off competition, the Red Cross designed and launched a hospital vendor discount program. "American Red Cross Preferred" was billed as a way for hospitals to lower their cost of doing business, although initially incurring greater expense. "[A] select collection of hospital suppliers" would offer special discounts for their products to hospitals that receive blood from the Red Cross *exclusively*. Such discounts would extend to medical equipment, consulting, pharmaceuticals, insurance, and disposables. "These discounts," the marketing plan stated, "should ultimately allow ARC customers to save money . . . even though some ARC products may be more expensive."

Such a "creative strategy" would, headquarters predicted, "play a critical role in maintaining a competitive status until the cost reduction initiatives take effect. Further, this should be virtually impossible for competitors to respond to." So staggering were its implications and potential liabilities that the Red Cross Preferred option was rejected by attorneys from several pharmaceutical firms which had been approached.

Since the late 1980s, the Red Cross donor recruitment had been declining one to three percent per year. Donor acquisition was key to obtaining product. But recruitment and blood collection also represented Red Cross's highest costs. The idea was to cut those costs while increasing product. Headquarters' solution was to devise a plan by which its local disaster relief chapter would act as an entry point for donor recruitment in non–Red Cross blood regions. Blood Services could then export that local blood to regions where its own recruitment lagged. That blood could also be sold to hospitals in other areas where higher prices could be had.

Red Cross disaster relief chapters had, historically, functioned largely autonomously. Many, like the disaster chapter in Oklahoma City, also processed tissue and bone products, a lucrative side business. The Oklahoma City chapter had an amicable agreement with Oklahoma Blood Institute to use its labs for tissue testing. However, such community arrangements did not figure into headquarters' vision. Headquarters' plan was to establish "collaborative relationships" between disaster relief chapters and Red Cross Blood Services.

In anticipation of resistance from chapters, the Board of Governors empowered headquarters to override objections to this new National policy by local chapters. Should a chapter refuse to cooperate, the Blood Services region could appeal to headquarters to intervene. The board determined, "Corporate management [also] has the authority to determine whether chapter agreements with non–Red Cross blood collection entities are in conflict with the best interests of the American Red Cross, and if so, to instruct the chapter(s) to end such agreements." Thus, existing agreements between chapters and non–Red Cross blood banks could be arbitrarily severed at the discretion of headquarters.

Elizabeth Dole was also leveraging her and her husband's political clout to recruit donors en masse. In Marietta, Georgia, home of Lockheed Martin—whose CEO, Norm Augustine, was Red Cross's board chairman, the Red Cross circulated a "Dear blood donor" letter among employees. The letter encouraged the plant workers to "save your blood donations for the Red Cross." Marietta had long been served by the Florida-based Civitan community blood bank.

When in February, Mrs. Dole secured a million-dollar annual service commitment to the Red Cross from Federal Express, a supporter of Bob Dole, she also won the exclusive right to conduct blood drives among the 24,000 employees at the company's Memphis, Tennessee headquarters. The Red Cross had supplied less than two percent of the blood needed by Memphis hospitals, which were served by Lifeblood, a community blood bank consortium. At about that time, the Red Cross also signed a contract naming Federal Express its sole overnight carrier.

In one of its own regions, the Red Cross managed to score a 17,000-pints-a-year coup. The Chesapeake-Potomac blood bank struck a deal with Walter Reed Army Medical Center, making the Army base accessible for its frequent blood drives. In exchange, the Army received one credit for each pint of red blood which soldiers donated to the Red Cross. When Walter Reed needed blood, it could cash in those credits at a rate of one-to-one for red blood and two-to-one for platelets.

Mrs. Dole's more ambitious plan to corner the entire U.S. military as an exclusive Red Cross donor pool met with less success. Along with other community blood banks, the Red Cross had limited access to that coveted donor pool. Mrs. Dole attempted to change that equation. On February 6, Red Cross's Anthony Polk, former head of the Armed Forces Blood Program, contacted his successor, Lieutenant Colonel Michael J. Ward. Polk conveyed to Ward his new boss's desire to gain exclusive rights to conduct Red Cross blood drives at military bases nationwide. Mrs. Dole wanted the same exclusivity applied to human organs and tissue.

Ward suggested that Mrs. Dole contact the Assistant Secretary of Defense, Dr. Stephen C. Joseph. Subsequently, Red Cross senior vice president Jimmy Ross wrote Joseph asking for a meeting. Ward and other senior officials objected. Nonetheless, the meeting took place on April 26 between Jimmy Ross and Dr. Joseph. In an internal memo disclosed by the *New York Times*, Ward wrote, "The plot thickens. The Senate Armed Services Committee asked Dr. Joseph . . . very pointed questions regarding ARC-DOD [Department of Defense] relationships. Now I see why Dr. Joseph wouldn't cancel the meeting. This is very political."

Mrs. Dole would not receive an answer from Assistant Secretary Joseph until the summer of 1996, when he would decide there was no compelling reason to change the military's existing arrangements allowing multiple blood banks access.

She did manage to secure a new deal with the military. The Red Cross had long provided a free communications service between military personnel abroad and their loved ones at home. Not anymore. The government would now have to pay $43.5 million over the next three years for that service—this in addition to the $14.5 million already allocated to the Red Cross through the Defense Business Operations Fund of the Department of Defense.

In its continuing efforts to draw in donors, the Red Cross was offering community blood banks an opportunity to join its "Affiliation Program." That plan promised local blood banks national support, including, rather ironically, a "National Donor Recruitment Program," but with "local focus, identity, and control."

The Red Cross had also converted its 1993 Consent Decree for Permanent Federal Injunction into a selling point. According to its marketing materials, the organization's legal obligation under court mandate to finally comply with blood safety laws became the "FDA-approved quality assurance program." Its Charles Drew Institute training program was described as state-of-the-art industry education. "Standardized operating procedures, training and equipment, Total Quality Program, [and] centralized information systems"—all of which had been court ordered—became programs endorsed by the FDA.

A release quoted Steve Stachelski, Red Cross's vice president for Quality Assurance, as saying, "The [FDA] acceptance of our [Quality Assurance] plan is a tribute to the openness of the regular dialogue we have established with FDA on this and other matters." Senior vice president Jimmy Ross referred to FDA's approval as evidence of "the wisdom of our Transformation program."

The Affiliation Program plan was a hard sell. Only a few community banks had signed on. As the Council of Community Blood Centers executive director Jim MacPherson observed, "Why would anyone want to come on board an act that can't get itself together?"

In 1995 alone, several incidents raised questions as to the quality of Red Cross products.

In March, the Red Cross voluntarily withdrew over fifty lots of plasma derivatives—potentially as much as 400,000 individual blood products—manufactured from a donor suspected of having Creutzfeldt-Jacob Disease (CJD), an untreatable degenerative neurological disorder that causes dementia and death. This recall occurred soon after an earlier withdrawal of tens of thousands units of plasma products from two donors confirmed to have CJD.

By May 1995, more than $53 million worth of Red Cross plasma products were on hold.

One of the largest recalls occurred in April 1995, at the Red Cross's Greater Cleveland Center. The center announced a voluntary recall of 75,000 blood products due to defective hepatitis-B testing. It had gone undetected in these products for more than two years despite notification by the manufacturer of glitches in the computer software in testing back in September 1992. The *Cleveland Plain Dealer* reported that the Red Cross could not determine which of the 450,000 units of blood it sold to area hospitals during that time had been improperly screened for the disease.

Yet the Red Cross claimed in a press release: "Thanks to one of the most sophisticated computer systems in the Blood Services industry, the Red Cross has been able to quickly select and recall only those units affected by the malfunction." A few months later the Red Cross said its recall was a false alarm.

FDA inspection reports identified nearly 80,000 units of Red Cross blood that had been recalled since 1993 because of faulty testing for HIV, hepatitis, syphilis, and bacterial contaminations and acceptance of blood from donors with a history of cancer and other problems.

Many of the CCBC's seventy-two blood banks solicited by the Red Cross for its Affliation Program were more than reluctant to join; they were outraged. The program ran counter to the National Blood Policy Act, which the Red Cross had supported in the late 1970s. That voluntary policy was created following congressional hearings on blood shortages; its purpose was to protect the integrity of local blood bank management and prevent the kind of donor recruitment skirmishes the Red Cross was now inciting. CCBC president Dr. Toby Simon expressed his constituents' concerns to Norman Augustine. In a November 5, 1995 letter, Simon wrote, "The Red Cross has either forgotten or has chosen to ignore and abandon the National Blood Policy. If the latter, it has done so without consulting Congress, the Department of Health and Human Services, or the communities we all serve. That policy, which the Red Cross once both championed and embodied, empowers a national system of community-based and managed blood centers, many of which have held the public trust for over fifty years." Simon told Augustine, "There's strong evidence that volunteer donors will not support such a use of their gift. I fear that widespread disillusionment by the donors will lead to serious blood shortages."

Attorneys for Red Cross responded, declining to enter into a discussion about the issues Simon had raised.

CHAPTER NINETEEN

MORAL STANDARDS

*We won't survive as a nation if we don't recognize certain
overriding truths—in other words, moral standards.*

Elizabeth Dole
May 1995

The presidential primary season swung into action with candidates
hurriedly factoring in a formidable political sector. The 1.5 million
member Christian Coalition was comprised largely of hard core religious activists and social conservatives. It had been a significant
force during the so-called November, 1994 "Republican Revolution"
which hurled scores of vocal young conservatives into Congress.
Conservative support would, political analysts recognized, be key to
winning the upcoming Republican presidential primaries in Iowa,
New Hampshire and throughout the South.

The issues that resonated with this group included: "family values," school prayer, bans on abortion, gay rights, sex education and
AIDS prevention programs.

Although Bob Dole was a bona fide fiscal conservative, his voting
record on social issues was not particularly attractive to the Christian Right. Dole had supported civil rights legislation and opposed
all types of discrimination, including against homosexuals. He was
a proponent of affirmative action, AIDS research and some social
welfare programs like food stamps and school lunches. He rarely
spoke of moral values, favoring instead discussions about budget
deficits and legislative process, God and marriage were his wife's do-
main. In early 1995, Rev. Patrick Mahoney, head of the traditional

values Christian Defense Coalition pegged Dole as a "country club Republican" with little interest in any of the "core issues" important to evangelicals and pro-family activists.

"There's no question about it," Dole countered. "I'm not perceived as being hard right. I don't want to be perceived as hard right. If that's what it takes to win the nomination, it won't happen to me."

During his 1988 campaign, Bob Dole had written off support from the religious right, since TV evangelist Pat Robertson, founder of the Christian Coalition, was himself in the race. But in the 1996 challenge, Dole's opponents Pat Buchanan and Texas Senator Phil Gramm conversed easily on the topics of morality, family and church. Neither had, however, yet wrapped up the Christian vote.

Pushing Dole hardest to the right was Mrs. Dole's politically astute protégé, Mari Maseng-Will. In late 1994, Mrs. Dole had called in Maseng-Will to render an assessment of issues surrounding her husband's third presidential bid. Mrs. Dole's Red Cross Special Teamer rolled over to the Republican campaign and was named Bob Dole's director of communications and speech writer. Special Team colleague John Heubusch had already departed from the Red Cross, where he was vice president for communications, to become executive director of the National Republican Senatorial Campaign Committee.

The message Maseng-Will penned was designed to affiliate Dole, intellectually and spiritually, with the Christian Right. His speeches in Kansas, Iowa and New Hampshire were peppered with appeals for "a return to fundamental values." He attacked drug dealers and welfare mothers, and advocated an end to the affirmative action programs he had once supported. He urged passage of an amendment to allow voluntary school prayer. In one of Maseng-Will's most flamboyantly written orations, Dole blasted Hollywood for the "mainstreaming of deviance," and its productions that were "nightmares of depravity."

As her husband's "partner unlimited," Elizabeth Dole had proven herself adept at sidestepping political minefields and steering his monied supporters her way. Her timely, seemingly seamless rebirth of faith, had them switching their house of worship from the socially moderate Foundry Methodist to traditional Evangelical. In the spring of 1995, she began combining travel as Red Cross president with inspirational speeches, at prayer breakfasts, guest appearances and gatherings like the "God and Country Rally" sponsored by the

Christian Coalition in Florida. She told audiences that she began "each new journey Life brings with a prayer." To a Christian high school commencement crowd she explained, "God does not want worldly successes—he wants your heart in submission to His will. . . . "Life is not just to spend a few years on career . . . [it's] a stewardship to be lived according to a much higher calling."

But when the Christian Right directed its moral compass at the Red Cross, Mrs. Dole's maneuvering had to be far more dexterous. Just how well she met that challenge became a fiercely debated topic.

Ever since she assumed presidency of the Red Cross, the cross fertilization of personnel and finances between the Doles had become more pronounced. By 1995, big money contributors were sorely needed to blacken the Red Cross's red ink. The organization's fiscal portfolio looked bleak. Headquarters and Blood Services regions were expecting to end fiscal '95 with a deficit of $76 million in Biomedical Services. That projection reflected $27 million more in the regions and $16 million more at headquarters than had been originally budgeted. Biomedical Services would, in fact, post a $113.4 million deficit in fiscal 1995. The Red Cross attributed its deficit to regulatory holds on significant amounts of plasma derivative products, one of its largest revenue sources; mounting operating costs in the Blood Services regions; and continued investments in Transformation. Although much of the plasma had since been released for sale, the year-long freeze had weakened the Red Cross market share for selected products and put a crimp in customer relations. Blood regions suffered from declining donations and continued costs involving centralization. Administrative and support functions in the various regions had not been fully consolidated.

For the first time, Biomedical Services had to borrow from the Disaster Relief Fund. That $12.8 million loan was, headquarters said, taken from the part of the Disaster Relief Fund controlled by the board—not from donor-restricted contributions. Biomedical borrowed another $34 million from other chapter operations funds. As to the impact of such borrowing, headquarters told the regions, "The most serious consequence was its effect on national sector cash flow." Headquarters assured the areas the Red Cross was not in immediate danger of lacking cash to pay for operating costs, payroll, or disaster relief expenses.

To address the money crunch, headquarters was forging what internal documents described as "strategic alliances that are revenue producing." The model on which these joint ventures was based was the Red Cross's Federal Express partnership, which enhanced both the charity's financial picture and its donor pool. Along those lines, the Red Cross conceived its most ambitious venture: "Rx for Life." A loose consortium of 14 research-based pharmaceutical companies, "Rx for Life" would not only donate $20 million to the Red Cross but help recruit new donors through a national media, telemarketing, and direct mail program.

Bob Dole had long been favored among the pharmaceutical and health care products industry. In 1995, thirty-seven major pharmaceuticals supported his presidential aspirations, either through direct individual contributions or through selected political action committees. Nine of "Rx for Life's" fourteen members were among those political backers.

Other prospects for joint ventures were on the horizon in the areas of information systems and medical supplies. Information Data Management for the development and implementation of a nationwide computing system and infrastructure to support standardized applications; Baxter Healthcare Corporation, to develop and supply high-tech blood bags, plasma fractionation, and blood processing equipment; and Johnson & Johnson, for hospital laboratory/blood bank/transfusion service management. In the biotechnology arena, the Red Cross was looking to enter the blood products substitute market with Baxter Healthcare Corporation, Northfield Laboratories, and Upjohn Company. In the area of biotech safety and product development, appealing partners were Hemasure, Genzyme, and Osteotech.

The Red Cross also gained access to another of Bob Dole's backers, winery kingpins Ernest and Julio Gallo. The Center for Public Integrity described the Gallo family as Bob Dole's "most generous patron." With contributions totaling more than $1.4 million since 1979, the billion-dollar-a-year winery and the extended Gallo family have written checks for $381,000 to Dole's campaigns and political action committees, contributed $100,000 to his now-defunct think tank, the Better America Foundation, and supported the Dole Foundation for Employment of People with Disabilities to the tune of $790,000. In return, Dole had been responsible for the passage of what became known as the "Gallo amendment." That provision gave substantial tax breaks to inheritances within large families like the Gallos. Dole successfully lobbied the Treasury Department's Bureau of Alcohol and Firearms to give Gallo a waiver from labeling regulations, and in 1994, he answered President Clinton's health care initiatives with specific exclusions of "sin taxes" on alcohol and tobacco.

In 1995, the vintners extended their largesse to Dole's wife through a $100,000 cash contribution to the American Red Cross. As former Dole financial adviser David Owen observed on *Frontline*, "In the case of Bob and Elizabeth Dole, she's such a public person and such a powerhouse in her own right, when they help her, I think they believe that they're helping him."

Such business donations to the Red Cross were relatively straightforward. They might involve the appointment of a generous donor's spouse to the board or a sales plug for a corporate donor. Still, there had been no need for concessions to a donor's particular agenda. When the Christian Right gained early access to Red Cross's revised AIDS education material, the payback equation changed.

The Red Cross had been granted $5 million in federal funding from the Centers for Disease Control to update the organization's ten-year-old AIDS education program. "AIDS 101," as it was referred to, developed into a multilevel, multifaceted awareness package that included a manual, posters, leaflets, and a video. A collaborative effort among public health experts, educators, and physicians, the presentation was direct and nonjudgmental. By spring, the largest AIDS education program in the United States had been focus group–tested and approved internally at the Red Cross. Colleges, churches, civic groups, and all Red Cross centers and chapters were awaiting delivery.

Months went by—still no materials. The regions began asking questions. Headquarters was evasive.

In early September, Jim Graham, an attorney and longtime executive director of the Whitman-Walker Clinic, received a call from a friend at the Red Cross. The clinic, named for the poet Walt Whitman and Civil War surgeon Dr. Mary Walker, was the primary provider of the community-based medical and social services for people with AIDS in the Washington, D.C. area. Graham could hear the anxiety in his friend's voice. Mrs. Dole was withholding the AIDS education materials. There was some concern about the drawing of testicles being too explicit, and about the graphic depiction of the placement of condoms. There was not enough emphasis on abstinence.

In an extraordinary move, the Board of Governors had created a special committee to review the materials. The board had never before been involved in those kinds of decisions.

Graham's contact told him something big was going on. He wanted him to go to the *New York Times*.

The clinic director asked to see the materials first. That was out of the question, he was told; they could not leave headquarters. Graham felt uncomfortable about making the press call, but he became obsessed with getting a look at the withheld materials. He plugged into his AIDS information network and subsequently received the controversial Red Cross material. The drawings in question were childlike, almost cartoons.

The *New York Times* story ran on September 13, apparently leaked by another source. By then Graham had pieced together the attendant politics. As he saw it, the partisan consideration had superseded an important public health issue.

The scenario that would emerge over the subsequent months centered, not surprisingly, on campaign politics. The Christian Right group Americans for Sound AIDS/HIV policy, (ASAP) had managed a preview of the Red Cross's AIDS package. It was not pleased. Several members of the Special Team suggested she reexamine the materials and Mrs. Dole delayed publication. In a highly unusual move, she asked the Board of Governors to step in and neutralize the material to place greater emphasis on abstinence and "individual responsibility," a catch phrase appropriated by the conservative right.

Red Cross personnel at the chapters were outraged. One AIDS-education coordinator whose region was experiencing a surge in AIDS among teens had assumed the hold-up was political. "Until Mrs. Dole or the people on the Board of Governors have stood by as many graves as I have," she said angrily, "I don't think they have a right to tell me how to do my job."

Shortly after the news broke, Graham received another call from his Red Cross contact. He was told that heads would roll.

In an attempt to downplay the political inference, the organization swiftly issued a policy statement: "Mrs. Dole asked the board to become involved in order to ensure there would be no false perception that politics had entered into the issues."

In an effort at further damage control, officials distributed an agency-wide memo accusing the *New York Times* of distortions and blaming unnamed Red Cross chapter officials for the press leak. The memo also advised staff how to publicly defend the program's revision.

In a September 16 press conference, Red Cross's president attempted to distance herself from the controversy, vigorously denying that she had requested changes in the AIDS material to protect her husband's appeal to conservative voters. "I recommended to the chairman of the American Red Cross that the board handle the issue." Mrs. Dole said of her contact with Chairman Norman Augustine. "It's very obvious that I didn't want to have any possible question about politics or I would have just done it myself. But I turned it over to the Board." She added, "I didn't have anything to do with that." Bob Dole defended his wife: "My view is that Elizabeth has been very scrupulous in keeping politics out of it."

Mrs. Dole, who had managed to escape unscathed from controversies that plagued her role in several presidential administrations, was vilified in news reports, editorials, and commentaries.

After being significantly changed, the AIDS education materials were subsequently released.

Five days after the *Times* story, Mrs. Dole announced her decision to take a leave of absence from the Red Cross. In a statement issued by Bob Dole's campaign headquarters, his wife said, "I'm leaving now to help my husband. I hope one day to help him as First Lady. But I'll always be a Red Crosser. I'll be back." She asked the Board to grant her a leave of absence.

While Mrs. Dole was awaiting the board's decision, Donna Shalala, Secretary of Health and Human Services, took an unprecedented step. She appointed a federal manager to oversee the safety of the nation's blood supply. The appointee, Philip Lee, Assistant Health Secretary, would "facilitate leadership and give priority to blood safety issues at the highest level during times of crisis and disagreement." Shalala also created a Blood Safety Council, which included experts from the CDC, the FDA, and the NIH. The designation of these watchdogs was in response to a report issued months earlier by the Institute of Medicine (IOM).

The IOM issued a report in July 1995, entitled "HIV and the Blood Supply: An Analysis of Crisis Decisionmaking." It was the culmination of a year-long study, commissioned by Secretary Shalala, of the events that led to the contamination of the blood supply by HIV in the early 1980s. The report was prepared by a committee of scholars, ethicists and medical experts in the fields of public health, blood banking and communicable disease. They examined the decisions made between 1982 through 1985 to safeguard blood and blood products. The committee interviewed dozens of government and blood industry officials, including Drs. Gerald Sandler, Leon Hoyer, and Peter Page, of the Red Cross and former Red Cross counsel Karen Shoos Lipton, who had since become head of the American Association of Blood Banks. The committee also took public testimony from scores of witnesses.

The report found that by January 1983, strong evidence existed to indicate that AIDS was transmissible through blood. However, blood banks, plasma manufacturers and FDA chose a "very cautious" approach that subjected them to "a minimum of criticism."

Preference for the "status quo" led many in the blood banking industry to underestimate the threat of transfusion AIDS. "Blood bank officials and federal authorities consistently chose the least aggressive option that was justifiable. In adopting this limited approach, policy makers often passed over options that might have initially slowed the spread of HIV to individuals with hemophilia and other recipients of blood and blood products," the report said. It concluded, "The Committee believes it was reasonable to require blood banks to implement these two screening procedures [direct donor questioning and surrogate blood testing] in January 1983," and that such measures "probably would have reduced the number of individuals infected with HIV through blood and blood products."

The IOM findings confirmed what plaintiffs in transfusion-AIDS cases had been telling the courts for a decade: that the entities responsible for the U.S. blood system—from the federal government to for-profit plasma manufacturers to community blood banks and the American Red Cross—failed in the 1980s to ensure the safety of the blood supply.

Two weeks after Shalala's announcement of the appointment of federal blood watchdogs, the Board of Governors of the Red Cross granted Mrs. Dole an unpaid leave of absence for approximately one year, after which she fully expected to return to the Red Cross as the only First Lady in history to have a full-time job.

In a prepared statement, Elizabeth Dole said of her time at the Red Cross, "Of all my challenges in public service, this one provides perhaps the greatest satisfaction, offering disaster relief to literally tens of thousands of victims throughout the world and helping to ensure the continued safety and availability of the nation's blood supply . . . I have a continuing concern for at-risk youth, and I believe, both as First Lady and president of the Red Cross, I could help the country rekindle its spirit of volunteerism and philanthropic giving."

When her sister Hailey talked about going to heaven, what color it would be (Heather had said it was purple, Hailey insisted it was pink), Holly would change the subject or walk into another room. When Hailey died at age ten in the spring of 1994, Holly absorbed herself in her schoolwork. She earned straight A's, even A+'s. Her classmates, who adored her, nicknamed her "Wonder Woman." She always had a ready smile.

On Christmas Day, Holly told her grandmother about a dream she had had the previous night. "The lights were blinking on the tree and I looked up and it was Hailey, and she says 'It's me, Holly! I want you to know I am okay. I'm fine. Don't worry, be happy. I'm always gonna be watching over you and Granny.' " On New Year's Day 1995, Holly wrote a story and gave it to her grandmother. She titled it "Cure."

My New Year's resolution is to help find a cure for all the diseases like AIDS, Lukemia [sic], and all of the rest of the bad diseases. What makes me mad is that every person who has AIDS, Cancer or any other very bad disease, they usually end up dying. But I believe in true miracles. You've got to have a lot of strength, courage, hope, prayers and faith in yourself. Maybe, just maybe, one day they will find a cure for all the bad diseases.

By then, Holly had lost most of her sight. "It's like I'm looking through a straw, Granny," she explained. In late October, she was confined to a wheelchair. One quiet wintry night, she was listening to Mariah Carey. Jewelle Ann was beside her, crocheting. "You know, Granny," Holly suddenly said, "we're not really in this body when we leave."

On November 9, Jewelle Ann Michaels had a dream. "I'd seen all of them," she would later recall. "They were tap dancing. They had their hair up. They were dancing and singing. 'Do you like it, Granny?' they asked me. They were laughing and tapping and fading away. I said, 'Come back!' Then all three of them started waving and calling out to me, with those pretty doll-baby smiles, 'Don't worry, Granny. Be happy.' Then they faded away."

Holly died that night. She was eleven years old.

APPENDIX I: CHARTS

WHAT BLOOD IS

Always considered a mysterious, magical fluid, blood is actually composed of many different types of cells all suspended in a pale yellow fluid called plasma. It circulates throughout the body through the pumping action of the heart and is carried through blood vessels called arteries and veins. Its main functions are to transport oxygen, hormones, and vital nutrients to every cell of the body and to carry away wastes. Blood helps regulate body temperature, as well as fluid and salt balance. It also protects against disease by carrying antibodies that recognize any foreign agent, or pathogen, that manages to invade the body. Testing blood samples help chemistry levels and other factors to evaluate the presence or absence of disease.

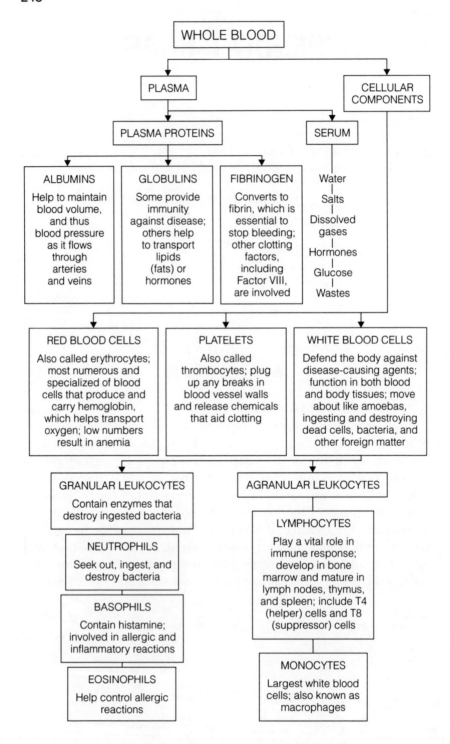

FRACTIONATION

Fractionation is the process of breaking blood plasma down into special products, each of which has a unique part to play in the treatment of diseases and disorders. The process was discovered during World War II and the demand since then for plasma now exceeds the demand for other cellular parts of blood. Most of these products are derived from donations by many thousands of people who contribute to a "plasma pool." Screening tests are necessary to ensure that blood is not contaminated to prevent the spread of disease. The main products of plasma are shown below.

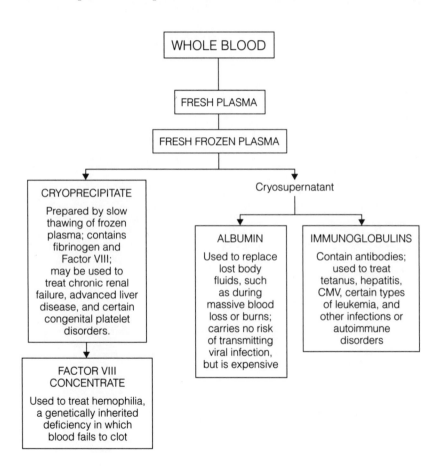

GLOSSARY

Entries in *italics* are cross-referenced.

AABB: American Association of Blood Banks. A major *blood banking* organization, and a trade group that helps set blood bank standards.

AIDS: Acquired Immunodeficiency Syndrome. A disease in which the body's immune system breaks down and is unable to deal with infections that, in a normal person, the body can resist. Usually fatal within two to ten years of infection with the human immunodeficiency virus *(HIV)*. Sources of transmission include infected or contaminated blood and blood products, unsterile needles (usually shared by drug abusers), and semen; the virus can also be transmitted in utero from a woman to her fetus. Symptoms include weight loss, *opportunistic infections, Kaposi's sarcoma, lymphadenopathy,* and neurological disorders. Currently treated by certain drugs, such as *AZT.* As yet there is no vaccine and no cure.

Albumin: the most abundant protein in the body, which forms part of blood plasma. Certain hormones and drugs circulating in the blood bind to molecules of albumin so that they are not excreted by the kidney. As a byproduct of *fractionation,* albumin isolated from plasma is used to maintain blood volume and pressure, especially in the treatment of severe burns and shock.

Anemia: a blood disorder that causes pallor, breathlessness, dizziness, and heart palpitations. It is caused by the reduced or impaired production, or excessive destruction, of red blood cells. Normally, these cells contain a pigment known as *hemoglobin,* a molecule to which oxygen binds. A low concentration of hemoglobin reduces the oxygen-carrying capacity of the blood. There are many types and causes of anemia; most commonly it is due to iron deficiency (iron is a necessary component of hemoglobin), but anemia can also be caused by loss of blood from heavy menstrual periods or internal bleeding.

Antibody: a protein produced by one type of white blood cell (B-lymphocytes, which develop in the lymph nodes) as part of the body's immune response. Antibodies form in response to invading foreign proteins *(antigens)* that are contained in bacteria, viruses, and other microorganisms. When disease threatens, antibodies that are specifically formed circulate in the bloodstream and body tissues in order to target and destroy the antigens. Antibodies are known as *immunoglobulins.*

Antigen: protein or carbohydrate substance that when introduced into the body stimulates the production of an antibody.

Antihemophilic Factor: a blood protein found in *plasma,* also known as AHF, Factor VIII, or antihemophiliac globulin. It is essential for blood *coagulation* (the process by which blood solidifies and form clots). The absence of this protein, due to a defective *gene,* causes *hemophilia.*

Apheresis: a method of collecting specific components of blood, such as *platelets* or *plasma,* instead of whole blood. It takes about two and a half hours.

Autologous transfusion: a transfusion used in *elective surgery,* in which the person's own blood is used. The blood will have been collected before the surgery, and specifically reserved for the patient's own use.

AZT: the abbreviation for azidothymidine, formerly called *zidovudine* (ZDV). An antiviral drug (one that inhibits the replication of viral molecules), it was the first medication approved by the FDA in the treatment of patients who are HIV positive but have no symptoms of AIDS; it also appears to increase the survival time of those with full-blown AIDS.

Bleeding: loss of blood caused by damage to blood vessels, usually through injury. Blood loss is not only visible (outside the body): concealed (internal) blood loss can occur if internal organs or blood vessels are injured, infected, or inflamed. Bruising occurs when blood collects beneath the skin. Excessive blood loss may result in shock (faintness, sweating, pallor) or death.

Blood: a sticky red fluid carried in a complex network of arteries, veins, and capillaries. Specialized cells and proteins transport oxygen, nutrients, and hormones to body tissues and help to remove carbon dioxide and wastes.

Blood bank: a general term to describe a facility where blood and blood components are stored and later distributed. Such facilities may be part of a hospital or at an independent site; blood collection and processing may occur at a blood bank or at another location.

Blood center: a facility that collects, tests, processes, and distributes blood and blood products.

Blood donation: the giving of blood, which will be used by oneself or by someone else. Whole blood is usually given and will be broken down into components later, although it is now possible to extract components as well (see *apheresis*). A donation, which usually involves taking a small blood sample, a medical history, and sometimes readings of pulse and blood pressure, takes about forty-five minutes.

Blood groups: the way blood is classified into groups depending on the proteins, or antigens, on the surface of red blood cells. These marker proteins are called A and B. If a person's blood contains one or the other antigen, it is classed as either A or B; if it contains both markers, it is type AB; if neither, it is classed as O. Blood to be transfused must match the patient's type. More than 400 other antigens have been identified, but these rarely cause problems during transfusion. Blood is also classified by its *Rh factor.*

Blood pooling: the process by which individual units of blood (or blood products), collected from more than one donor at more than one location, are grouped together to form a larger unit.

Blood products: a general term for the various components of blood, such as whole blood, plasma, and clotting factors, each of which has a specific use in blood transfusion. Many are created by *fractionation*.

Blood transfusion: the infusion of blood from an outside source directly into a person's bloodstream. Blood from a donor must be cross-matched—that is, compatible—with the recipient's blood type. The volume of blood varies according to how much blood has been lost. In certain cases, an exchange transfusion is performed, during which nearly all of a recipient's blood is replaced by donor blood.

B-lymphocytes: a type of white blood cell that produces *antibodies*. Beginning life in the bone marrow, B-lymphocytes develop in *lymph nodes*. Like a key fitting into a lock, each B cell produces a specific antibody that will destroy only a specific antigen. Stimulated to proliferate by *T-lymphocytes*.

CCBC: Council of Community Blood Centers. The smallest of the major American *blood banks* organizations.

CD4 and **CD8:** types of *T-lymphocytes*.

CDC: Centers for Disease Control. A federal organization located in Atlanta, Georgia. Its task is to monitor the incidence and spread of infectious diseases in the United States.

Coagulation: the process by which blood solidifies and bleeding slows down. It occurs when platelets release certain clotting chemicals. Certain *factors* in blood plasma must be present if coagulation is to occur.

Concentrates: blood cells or proteins separated out from either whole blood or blood plasma.

Core antibody: an antibody produced in response to a "core antigen," or protein that forms the internal structure of a virus. Tests for core antibody help identify the presence of a virus. For example, a blood test for hepatitis core antibody will indicate if a person has been exposed to viral hepatitis.

Cross-matching: a test to ensure blood compatibility. A sample of the recipient's blood is taken for identification; it is then mixed with donor blood and examined under a microscope to discover if the recipient's blood has any *antibodies* that would damage donor blood cells. The procedure usually takes less than one hour.

Cryoprecipitate: a substance rich in Factor VIII (or AHF), which remains after blood plasma has been frozen and subsequently thawed.

Directed donation: a procedure by which blood is donated, at the recipient's request, by specific individuals. Family and friends may be asked or may volunteer to donate blood; this specific collection is then the sole source of blood for the patient. Also known as "designated donation."

Elective surgery: operations that may be recommended to a patient, but are not necessarily urgent or medical emergencies. They can usually be arranged in consultation with a physician to choose a mutually convenient time so that *directed donations* or an *autologous transfusion* can be arranged.

ELISA: acronym for a type of blood test, the enzyme-linked immunosorbent assay. It detects the presence of antibodies to *HIV* in the blood and is thus one test for *AIDS*.

Factor: a component of blood plasma designated by a Roman numeral. Factor I is a soluble protein called fibrinogen; it triggers the formation of fibrin, whose molecules form long filaments and help to stop bleeding. Factor VIII and Factor IX, when absent, cause hemophilia A and hemophilia B.

FDA: Food and Drug Administration. A federal agency with the capacity to enforce laws designed to protect the health of the country against "impure and unsafe foods, drugs, and cosmetics, and other potential hazards." Below are a few of its many departments (from the Office of Federal Register, U.S. Government Manual 1995–96, Washington D.C., 1995, pp. 289–292):

- the Office of Policy, which directs and coordinates the agency's rulemaking activities and plans regulatory reforms;
- the Office of Operations, which "develops and administers all agency field operations" pertaining to drugs, food, medical devices, and cosmetics;
- the Office of Management of Systems *(OMS)*, which plays a major role in "resource planning, development, and evaluation activities";
- the Center for Drug Evaluation and Research, which develops administration policy about the "safety, effectiveness, and labeling of all drug products for human use, . . . reviews

and evaluates new drug applications, . . . and monitors the quality of marketed drug products through product testing, surveillance, and compliance programs";
* the Center for Biologics Evaluation and Research, which is the major focus for coordinating the AIDS program, including the evaluation of diagnostic tests.

FFP (fresh-frozen plasma): plasma that has been frozen after collection in order to preserve vital *coagulation* factors; used to treat bleeding disorders.

Fractionation: the process by which plasma is broken down into its many components, such as *immunoglobulins, albumin,* and all the clotting *factors;* also called plasma fractionation.

Gene: a short segment or unit of hereditary material contained within the nucleus of a cell. Every human cell nucleus has more than 50,000 different genes which influence growth, development, and functioning. Defective genes can cause malfunctioning, and may also be inherited, as in *hemophilia.*

Heat treatment: the exposure of pooled plasma products to heat in order to destroy any live viruses.

Hematology: the study of blood and blood diseases.

Hemophilia: a rare inherited bleeding disorder. Caused by a defective gene and usually affecting only males, it results in a deficiency of clotting Factor VIII (hemophilia A) or Factor IX (hemophilia B). In the United States, about 1 in 10,000 males has hemophilia A, and in about 75 percent of cases, there is a previous family history of the disease. Those affected bruise very easily; repeated internal bleeding into joints and accumulated scar tissue may result in stiff joints and limited movement. Preventive treatment of severe bleeding episodes can be accomplished by regular transfusion of Factor VIII; in case of injury, additional transfusions are required.

Hepatitis: inflammation of the liver due to several different causes, including several types of virus (which can be transmitted during blood transfusions), bacteria, and certain chemicals, including alcohol.

Hepatitis B core antibody test: a blood screening test that detects *antibodies* to the protein found in the core (center) of the hepatitis B virus. A positive result would indicate exposure to the virus.

HIV: Human immunodeficiency virus, which is the primary cause of *AIDS*. It is transmissible through blood and semen and destroys the body's CD4 lymphocytes (see *T-lymphocytes*), the cells that normally attack invading disease organisms. The virus was first isolated in 1983 at the Pasteur Institute by Luc Montaignier, who called it LAV (lymphadenopathy-associated virus). An almost identical virus was isolated by Robert Gallo at the National Institutes of Health in 1984; Gallo called his virus HTLV-III (human T-lymphocyte virus). In 1986, this virus was designated HIV (or HIV-1).

Immune system: the body's defense against illness and disease, comprising specific cells (such as *T-lymphocytes*) and blood proteins (such as *antibodies*), which attack invading viruses, bacteria, and fungi.

Immunodeficiency disorders: what happens when the immune system is "compromised" and cannot fight infection or destroy tumors. Such disorders may be inherited or, as in the case of AIDS, acquired. Symptoms include incomplete recovery, or a persistent or recurrent infection, that a healthy person could overcome.

Immunoglobulins: proteins found in blood plasma and tissue fluids. Also known as *antibodies*, immunoglobulins are produced by *B-lymphocytes*. They bind to and destroy invading microorganisms that cause disease.

Kaposi's sarcoma: a condition characterized by multiple malignant skin tumors; in full-blown AIDS, tumors also affect the gastrointestinal and respiratory tracts, causing difficulties in digestion, elimination, and breathing.

Look-Back program: a system whereby recipients of blood that had been donated by people who are HIV-positive are traced by blood banks.

Lymphadenopathy: disease of the *lymph nodes*.

Lymph nodes: masses of a special type of tissue covered by a fibrous capsule. Also known as lymph glands, they cluster in specific areas, notably under the arms and in the groin, and range in size from 1 to 20 mm. Spaces within the nodes contain scavenging white blood cells that ingest bacteria; the centers release lymphocytes that produce antibodies. Lymph nodes are connected by a system of channels called lymphatics. Swollen nodes usually indicate disease.

Lymphoma: a malignant tumor in one of the *lymph nodes.*

NIH: National Institutes of Health, a division of the U.S. Department of Health and Services.

OMS: Office of Management and Systems. Part of the *FDA* that develops program and planning strategy by analyzing and evaluating issues. It plays a role in agency administration and financial management, including budget, grants, and contracts, and supports program operations.

Opportunistic infections: infections, caused by microorganisms, which, in a healthy person with a strong *immune system,* would either not cause infection or disease, or result in symptoms mild and easy to overcome. People with an impaired immune system are very susceptible to these types of infection.

P24 antigen: the *core antigens* found in *HIV.* Its presence is used to diagnose infection with the virus.

Pathogen: any agent or microorganisms that causes disease.

Plasma: the straw-colored liquid portion of whole blood, which remains when all blood cells are removed. Its salt content is similar to seawater, and it contains many nutrients, proteins *(see factor),* gases, and wastes.

Plasma fractionation: see *fractionation.*

Platelets: a specific type of blood cell that is essential for blood clotting. Activated when they contact damaged blood vessel walls, platelets clump together and then release chemicals that stimulate other coagulation factors, such as *AHF.*

Pneumocystis carinii (PCP): a type of pneumonia caused by a microorganism that affects people with an impaired *immune system;* previously a rare lung infection, it became an important diagnostic sign of full-blown *AIDS* as the disease spread.

Rh factor: the classification of blood into "positive" or "negative." Named for experiments with Rhesus monkeys, this system is based on the presence of *antigens.* One, known as factor D, occurs in about 85 percent of people, who are then known as Rh-positive; in the remaining 15 percent, the antigen is lacking, and they are designated Rh-negative.

Screening: the use of tests and examination to separate individuals with a pathological condition, such as an infectious disease, from those who are well.

Surrogate markers: laboratory tests that attempt to detect one disease-causing agent by testing for the presence of another. It is a method of trying to predict the spread of a disease with waiting for the development of a specific test. For example, people who test positive for HIV will likely also test positive for hepatitis B core antibody.

T-lymphocytes: a special group of white blood cells that are part of the immune system. Unlike *B-lymphocytes,* they do not produce *antibodies.* They begin life in the bone marrow, then migrate to the thymus gland, where they mature; they then migrate to other body tissues to fight against any invading *pathogen.* There are two types. T8 suppressor cells (also known as CD8 cells) travel to and attach themselves to cells that the body recognizes as abnormal; they then secrete chemicals called lymphokines that kill the invaders. They are aided by T4 (or CD4) helper cells. It is the number of CD4 cells that is drastically reduced in people who have AIDS: A low T-cell count is an indication of impaired immunity.

Transfusion: see *blood transfusion.*

APPENDIX II

KEEPING BLOOD SAFE

Every twelve seconds, someone needs blood. In fact, one in ten hospital patients will need a blood transfusion, as will ninety percent of us at some point in our lives. So the safety of the public blood supply isn't a remote issue: It clearly affects you—or someone close to you—now and in the future. What can you do?

Insist on Safe Blood
You can do this by writing to your congressional representative, citing this book as the source of your concern. State that, as an American citizen, you believe you are entitled to safe public health care. Insist on the following:

- Donor education programs so that high-risk donors are discouraged from contaminating the blood supply.
- Policies to trace and screen out infected donors.
- Updated and appropriate computer networks.
- The development and implementation of tests to ensure blood safety.

Give Blood Yourself

If you are in good health, becoming a regular donor will ensure that the supply of safe blood is continually replenished. Unlike receiving blood, giving blood exposes you to absolutely no risk at all.

Be Your Own Donor

If you need a transfusion, the safest blood you can receive is your own. If you know that you're going to have an operation, you can arrange with your physician and the hospital to give donations, at least six weeks in advance. Receiving blood you have donated yourself is known as an autologous transfusion.

Bear in mind that you must be in reasonably good health to give blood. If you're anemic or already suffering from a bacterial or viral infection, or if you have cancer, your doctor may discourage you from doing this.

In another procedure, you can request your blood to be collected and recycled during the operation itself. As with an autologous transfusion, this procedure is not recommended for all types of surgery, nor is it available at all hospitals, but do discuss the possibility with your doctor.

Talk to Your Friends and Family

If they're fit and well, encourage them to become regular blood donors. If you know you need to have an operation, consider asking them to donate blood for your use only if their blood type matches yours. This is called a "designated donation."

APPENDIX III: DOCUMENTS

Curran, CDC. Re: "Potential Transmission of KS/OI by Blood or Blood Products"

7-9-82 Memo: William H. Foege to State and Territorial Epidemiologists. Re: "Pneumocystis Carinii Pneumonia among Patients with Hemophilia"

7-9-82 Memo: William H. Foege to Hemophilia Treatment Centers. Re: "Pneumocystis Carinii Pneumonia among Patients with Hemophilia"

7-9-82 Memo: William H. Foege to L. C. Hershberger, Cutter Laboratories. Re: "Pneumocystis Carinii Pneumonia among Patients with Hemophilia"

7-9-82 Letter: William H. Foege to Dr. Alfred Katz

7-9-82 Internal Memo: Dr. Roger Dodd to Dr. Alfred Katz

7-9-82 Memo: Harry M. Meyer, Director, National Center for Drugs and Biologics, FDA, to Manufacturers of Plasma Fractionation Products. Re: "Meeting Concerning Opportunistic Infections in Hemophilia A Patients"

7-9-82 Internal Memo: Roger Dodd to Alfred Katz, ARC. Re: "Transmissible Opportunistic Infection Syndrome"

7-14-82 Internal Memo: Charles Carman to NHF Chapter Presidents. Re: "Attached NHF Patient Alert #1"

7-19-82 NHF Medical Bulletin. Signed by Louis Aledort, M.D.

7-19-82 NHF Chapter Advisory #2. Re: "Pneumocystis Carinii Pneumonia"

7-21-82 Letter: Bruce L. Evatt to Virginia Donaldson

7-21-82 Letter: Bruce L. Evatt to Oscar Ratnoff

7-23-82 Newsletter: Council of Community Blood Centers

7-26-82 Memo: Daniel J. Cassidy, AABB, to the Board of Directors, Committee on External Affairs. Re: "Hemophiliacs Contract Unexplained Acquired Cellular Immunodeficiency (UACI)"

7-27-82 Draft Agenda, Letter to Participants, List of Invitees and Summary Report, for "The Open Meeting of the PHS

Committee on Opportunistic Infections in Patients with Hemophilia"

7-30-82   NHF Medical Bulletin #2: "Acquired Immune Deficiency Syndrome (AIDS)", in Hemophilia Newsnotes

8-12-82   Newsletter: Council of Community Blood Centers

8-13-82   Briefing: James W. Curran. Task Force on Acquired Immune Deficiency Syndrome (AIDS). Table attached: "Kaposi's Sarcoma, Pneumocystis Carinii Pneumonia, and other Opportunistic Infections—Cases Reported to CDC"

8-20-82   Briefing: James W. Curran. Task Force on Acquired Immune Deficiency Syndrome (AIDS)

8-30-82   Internal Memo: J. Hink to Lee Hershberger, Cutter Laboratories. Re: "AIDS, KS, and PCP"

8-31-82   Letter: Bruce L. Evatt to James T. Sgouris.

9-3-82   Briefing: James W. Curran. Task Force on Acquired Immune Deficiency Syndrome (AIDS)

9-17-82   Briefing: James W. Curran. Task Force on Acquired Immune Deficiency Syndrome (AIDS)

9-24-82   Briefing: James W. Curran. Task Force on Acquired Immune Deficiency Syndrome (AIDS)

9-24-82   Summary Minutes: FDA Blood Products Advisory Committee Meeting #4

9-28-82   Internal Memo: Dr. Harold Maryman to Dr. Jamieson

10-2-82   Minutes: NHF Medical and Scientific Advisory Council Meeting

10-12-82   Briefing: Acquired Immune Deficiency Syndrome (AIDS) by James W. Curran

10-25-82   Memo for the Record: Dr. Katz, Executive Director, Blood Services, American Red Cross

10-27-82   Internal Memo: Dr. Llewellys Barker to Dr. Alfred Katz

11-2-82   Letter: Charles J. Carman, Chairman of the Board and

Louis M. Aledort, Medical Co-Director, National Hemophilia Foundation to Lewellys Barker, V.P. American Red Cross

11-2-82   Letter: Charles J. Carman and Louis M. Aledort, National Hemophilia Foundation to Jack Ryan, V.P., Cutter Laboratories

11-12-82   Letter: James W. Curran to Alfred Katz, American Red Cross

11-15-82   Letter: Jack Ryan, Cutter Laboratories to Charles Carman and Louis Aledort, National Hemophilia Foundation

11-20-82   AABB NewsBriefs: Volume 5, No. 11—November/December edition.

11-22-82   Briefing: "Acquired Immune Deficiency Syndrome (AIDS)", by James W. Curran. Attachment, "Questions and Answers on Acquired Immune Deficiency Syndrome (AIDS)"

11-30-82   AABB NewsBriefs: Volume 5, No. 11—November/December edition.

12-2-82   Internal Memo: Dr. Alfred Katz to Arnie de Beaufort

12-4-82   Summary Minutes: FDA Blood Products Advisory Committee Meeting # 5—"Workshop on the Evaluation of Stored Red Blood Cells"

12-6-82   Briefing: "Acquired Immune Deficiency Syndrome (AIDS)", by James W. Curran

12-7-82   Internal Memo: Gil Clark to the Board of Directors, AABB. Re: "Blood Products Advisory Committee Meeting Pertaining to Decreasing the Infectivity of Factor VIII Concentrate and AIDS and the CDC Address to the Health Sub-Committee of the House Commerce and Energy Committee". Highlights attached.

12-7-82   Memo: Walter Dowdle, Director CID, to William Foege, Director, CDC. Re: "AIDS"

12-8-82   Letter: Alfred J. Katz, Executive Director, Blood Services, American Red Cross to James Curran

12-9-82   NHF Chapter Advisory #4—"Acquired Immune Deficiency Syndrome (AIDS) Update".

12-10-82   Newsletter: Council of Community Blood Centers

12-13-82   Internal Memo: Steven J. Ojala, Cutter Laboratories. Re: "AIDS and FDA"

12-14-82   Briefing: Acquired Immune Deficiency Syndrome (AIDS) by James W. Curran

12-16-82   ARC Letter: Peter L. Page, Chief Medical Director, Blood Services—Northeast Region, to Alfred Katz, Executive Director. Re: "Proposed AIDS policy attached"

12-17-82   Internal Memo: Joseph R. Bove to the Committee on Transfusion Transmitted Diseases, AABB. Re: "AIDS"

12-17-82   NHF and CDC Survey: Acquired Immune Deficiency Syndrome (AIDS) Among Patients Attending Hemophilia Treatment Centers (HTC's)

12-17-82   Memo: To Alpha Therapeutic Corporation Source Plasma Centers. Attachments.

12-20-82   Memo: To Alpha Therapeutic Corporation Affiliate Blood Banks

12-21-82   Hemophilia Information Exchange: "AIDS Update"— NHF Medical Bulletin #4 and Chapter Advisory #5, Re: "AIDS:—Implications Regarding Blood Product Use; Summary of National Hemophilia Foundation Activities"

12-21-82   Internal Memo: S. J. Ojala, Cutter Laboratories. Re: "More AIDS and FDA"

12-22-82   Internal Memo: Edward O. Carr, MT(ASCP)SBB, President, AABB to AABB Institution and Associate Institutional Members. Re: "Acquired Immune Deficiency Syndrome (AIDS)"

12-22-82   Letter: Clyde McAuley, Medical Director, Alpha Therapeutic Corporation, to Hemophilia Treatment Centers and Chapters. Re: "Acquired Immune Deficiency Syndrome (AIDS)"

12-27-82 Letter: Charles Carman, Louis Aledort and Alan Brownstein, National Hemophilia Foundation to Jack Ryan, VP, Cutter Laboratories.

12-28-82 Internal memo: J. Hink to K. Fischer, Cutter Laboratories. Re: "Acquired Immune Deficiency Syndrome (AIDS)"

12-29-82 Internal Memo: Ed Cutter to Jack Ryan, Carolyn Patrick, Wayne Johnson, Ralph Roussell, George Akin, Cutter Laboratories. Re: "AIDS"

1-1-83 News Release: Sonoma County Community Blood Bank, "Acquired Immune Deficiency Syndrome (AIDS)".

1-4-83 Notice of Meeting, List of Invitees, Agenda, Sign-in Sheet, Slides and Summary Report: Public Health Service Meeting held at the CDC in Atlanta—"Workshop to Identify Opportunities for Prevention of Acquired Immune Deficiency Syndrome".

1-1-83 Hemophilia Bulletin of the L.A. Orthopaedic Hospital. Re: Acquired Immunodeficiency Syndrome (AIDS) and Hemophilia.

1-6-83 Letter: Leon Hoyer, University of Connecticut to Jeffrey Koplan, CDC. Re: January 4th meeting

1-6-83 Internal Memo: Donald Francis to Jeffrey Koplan. Re: Opportunities for Eliminating Blood Donors at Risk for Transmitting AIDS.

1-6-83 Internal Memo: John Hink to Dr. K. Fischer et al., Cutter Laboratories. Re: January 4th Meeting.

1-6-83 Letter: James Pert to James Curran. Re: January 4th AIDS Meeting

1-6-83 Memo: Alfred Katz to all ARC Blood Centres

1-7-83 Letter: Jeffrey Davis to Jeffrey Koplan. Re: January 4th Meeting.

1-7-83 Newsletter: Council of Community Blood Centres

1-7-83 ABRA Memo: from Robert Reilly, "AIDS: Public Statements". Attachments: Working Draft Adopted by TTD

Committee of the AABB. Re: Acquired Immune Deficiency Syndrome (AIDS); Alpha Therapeutics Memoranda.

1-10-83   News Release: National Gay Task Force, "Representatives from NGTF and Gay Health Care Community Play Crucial Role in National Blood Policy Decision".

1-11-83   AIDS Slides for Dr. Foege.

1-11-83   Letter: Louis Aledort, National Hemophilia Foundation to Jeffrey Koplan. Re: January 4th CDC meeting

1-11-83   Letter: R.J. Ravenhold to Jeffrey Koplan

1-12-83   Internal Memo: Steve Ojala, Cutter Laboratories to W.F. Schaeffler et al. Re: CDC/AIDS Meeting in Atlanta.

1-12-83   Letter: Charles Carman, National Hemophilia Foundation to Jeffrey Koplan. Re: January 4th meeting.

1-13-83   Joint Statement: AABB, ARC and CCBC, "Joint Statement on Acquired Immune Deficiency Syndrome (AIDS) Related to Transfusion".

1-13-83   Letter: Charles J. Carman of NHF to Dr. Koplan

1-14-83   Memo: Kenneth Woods to CCBC Trustees. Re: Joint Statement on Acquired Immune Deficiency Syndrome Related to Transfusion.

1-14-83   AIDS Briefing prepared by James Curran.

1-14-83   NHF MASAC Recommendations: "Recommendations to Prevent AIDS in Patients with Hemophilia".

1-14-83   Agenda, List of participants and Summary of NHF/Industry Strategy Meeting on AIDS.

1-17-83   NHF Bulletin #5/Chapter Advisory #6—"AIDS: NHF Medical and Scientific Advisory Council Develops Position; NHF and Industry Meet".

1-24-83   Report to Board: Committee on Transfusion Transmitted Diseases

1-25-83   Internal Memo: Dr. Alfred Katz to Management Staff of AIDS Workgroup

1-25-83 Internal Memo: Summary of responses to Dr. Alfred Katz, re: AIDS

2-1-83 Internal Memo: Dr. Gerald Sandler to Arnie de Beaufort

2-1-83 Internal Memo: Dr. J.P. O'Malley to Arnie de Beaufort

2-5-83 Internal Memo: Dr. Paul Cumming to Arnie de Beaufort

3-4-83 ARC News Release: "Red Cross Takes Action on AIDS".

3-7-83 Memo: Edward Carr, to AABB Members. Re: AIDS. Attachment: Joint Statement of AABB, ARC, and CCBC— "Joint Statement on Prevention of AIDS Related to Transfusion".

3-8-83 Internal Memo: Johanna Pindyck to Donor Chairperson, New York Blood Center.

3-8-83 Memo: Johanna Pindyck et al. to Nursing Department Staff, New York Blood Center. Re: AIDS procedures at Donor Sites.

3-9-83 NHF Chapter Advisory #7: "Update: AIDS Related Developments".

3-9-83 Letter: James Curran to Kenneth Woods, New York Blood Center.

3-9-83 Internal Memo: Louise Chiotes to All Phlebotomy Staff, New York Blood Center. Re: Implementation of AIDS Procedure.

3-9-83 Memo: John Bennett, CID to George Hardy, CDC. Re: Alpha Thymosin Testing.

3-14-83 Internal Memo: John Hink to Steven Ojala et al. Re: American Blood Resources Assn. Meeting—Las Vegas, "A Summary of the More Significant Information Discussed".

3-15-83 Agenda, List of Attendees, and Summary of NIH, Division of Blood Diseases and Resources Conference— "Conference on AIDS".

3-15-83 Letter: Marietta Carr, Alpha Therapeutics to John Petricciani, FDA.

3-15-83   Telex: W.Y. Cobb, DMSS to A.B. Morrison, HPB. Re: Acquired Immune Deficiency Syndrome (AIDS).

3-24-83   FDA Memo: John Petricciani to All Establishments Collecting Human Blood for Transfusion. Re: "Recommendations To Decrease the Risk of Transmitting Acquired Immune Deficiency Syndrome (AIDS) from Blood Donors".

3-24-83   FDA Memo: John Petricciani to All Establishments Collecting Source Plasma (Human). Re: "Recommendations To Decrease the Risk of Transmitting Acquired Immune Deficiency Syndrome (AIDS) from Blood Donors".

3-24-83   FDA Memo: John Petricciani to All Licensed Manufacturers of Plasma Derivatives. Re: "Source Material Used to Manufacture Certain Plasma Derivatives".

3-25-83   DHHS News Release.

3-25-83   Internal Memo: S.J. Ojala to M.N. Sternberg, Cutter Laboratories. Re: AIDS Update

3-28-83   Memo for the Record: Walter Dowdle, CID. Re: Meeting of Outside Consultants on the Association of AIDS with Blood and Blood Products

3-30-83   Report: AABB Transfusion Transmitted Diseases Committee Interim Report to the Board.

3-31-83   AABB News Release: "American Association of Blood Banks Issues Recommendations on AIDS."

4-4-83   Memo: Edward Carr to AABB Members. Re: Standard Operating Procedures Relating for Acquired Immune Deficiency Syndrome.

4-5-83   Bulletin: AABB Government Affairs Update, "Office of Biologics Issues AIDS Recommendations; AABB Develops SOP's".

4-7-83   Memo: Dr. Dahlke to Dr. Sherwood re: Implementation of transmissal sheet #288

4-8-83   Letter: Edward Brandt to Virginia Apuzzo. Re: March 4th Policy Statement on AIDS.

4-8-83 Memo for the Record: Roger Dodd. Re: Interagency Technical Committee Working Group on Blood Resources and Substitutes. Agenda attached.

4-14-83 Memo: Vincent DeVita to NCI Staff. Re: Formation of the NCI-AIDS Task Force.

4-23-83 Memo: Dr. Pearl Toy to Red Cross Blood Services Central California Region, Staff

4-28-83 Memo: Jim Curran to Drs. Bennett, Dowdle, Evatt et al. Re: Meeting of Outside Consultants on the Association of AIDS with Blood and Blood Products on May 12, 1983.

5-11-83 NHF Medical Bulletin #7/Chapter Advisory #8—*"NHF Urges Clotting Factor Use be Maintained"*.

5-1-83 West Virginia Epi-Log: "Prevention of AIDS, Report of Interagency Recommendations"

5-12-83 Agenda, List of Attendees, and Summary of Meeting of Consultants, "AIDS and Blood and Blood Products" held at CDC. Attachments: Study: "Possible Transfusion Associated AIDS—Adult"; Tables: "AIDS Patients with History of Receipt of Blood Products: Composite Patient and Donor Information—Adults and Infants".

5-24-83 DHHS News Release: "Statement by Edward N. Brandt Jr., M.D. Assistant Secretary for Health".

6-6-83 Draft Summary Minutes: Meeting of Inter-organizational Ad Hoc Working Committee on AIDS, Memorial Blood Bank.

6-6-83 Memo: Dr. Pearl Toy to Red Cross Blood Services Central California Region, Staff

6-13-83 Memo: S.J. Ojala to W.F. Schaeffler et al. Re: FDA Recall Recommendation Meeting, June 9, 1983.

6-17-83 Memo: Dr. Mabel Stevenson, Tri State Regional RCBS to Hospital Pathologists re: AIDS and Directed Donations

6-22-83 ABC Press Release: "A Message to American Blood Commission Members About AIDS and Transfusion from William V. Miller, MD, President".

6-22-83   ARC, AABB CCBC Joint News Release. Attachment: "Joint Statement on Directed Donations and AIDS".

6-23-83   Memo: Edward Carr to AABB Institutional and Associate Institutional Members. Re: Joint Statement on Directed Donations.

6-27-83   News Release: Red Cross joint release re: selection of blood donors

6-28-83   Stanford University Blood Bank Bulletin: "AIDS: Answers to Common Questions", Stanford University Medical Center.

6-28-83   Memo: Dr. Stevenson to All Physicians, Pathologists and Administrators at Tri State Regional RCBS

7-1-83   Alpha Hemophilia Letter: "New Clues Minimize AIDS' Risk to Hemophiliacs".

7-1-83   DHSS Pamphlet: "Facts About AIDS".

7-1-83   Letter: William Hartin, Alpha Therapeutics to Steve Ojala, Cutter Laboratories.

7-5-83   Internal Memo: Dr. Alfred Katz to Gerald Sandler

7-12-83   Internal Memo: Dr. Perkins to all physicians and nurses, Irwin Memorial Blood Bank. Re: Interpretation of AIDS questions.

7-13-83   Minutes: May 4th Interagency Technical Committee Meeting

7-27-83   Internal Memo: Mary Rae to Managers of Cutter-Affiliated Plasma Centers. Re: AIDS Notice.

8-1-83   Internal Memo: Johanna Pindyck to Donor Chairperson, New York Blood Center. Re: AIDS, Blood Donation and Blood Transfusion. Attachments: CUE form; Pamphlet, "What you should know about AIDS".

8-1-83   Statement: Alan Brownstein, NHF to House of Representatives Intergovernmental Relations and Human Resources Subcommittee of the Committee on Governmental Operations, "Hemophilia and Acquired Immune Deficiency Syndrome (AIDS): The Federal Response".

8-1-83   Statement: Joseph Bove on AIDS and Blood Transfusion Before the Intergovernmental Relations and Human Resources Sub-Committee of the Committee on Government Operations.

8-5-83   Bulletin: AABB Government Affairs Update.

8-23-83 Hemophilia Information Exchange: "AIDS: Acquired Immune Deficiency Syndrome: Questions and Answers".

8-23-83 Memorandum and Summary: Meeting of Consultants— AIDS and Blood and Blood Products, CDC, May 12, 1983.

8-26-83 Internal Memo: R.J. Modersbach to G. Akin, N. Ashworth, M. Budinger, R. Rousell, R. Schwartz, Cutter Laboratories. Re: AIDS Scenarios

8-29-83 Report: from AIDS Activity, CID, CDC: "Acquired Immunodeficiency Syndrome (AIDS): Weekly Surveillance Report".

8-31-83 Internal Memo: Dr. Gerald Sandler to Dr. Alfred Katz

9-2-83   Internal Memo: R. Barden to Dr. Rousell, Cutter Laboratories. Re: AIDS.

9-7-83   NHF Chapter Advisory #9 (Revised), "NHF Urges that Product Recall Should Not Change Use of Clotting Factor".

12-19-83 Internal Memo: Cutter Labs re: Anti-core testing

1983   Pamphlet: Red Cross Information, An Important message to All Blood Donors

1-1-84   Pamphlet: ARC, "What you should know about giving blood".

1-3-84   Letter: Alfred Katz to Barker, Wick and Schubert, ARC. Re: AIDS Status

1-3-84   Memorandum: Alfred Katz to Executive Heads, Directors and Medical/Scientific Directors. Re: AIDS update

1-3-84   Joint Statement: American Red Cross, American Association of Blood Banks and Council of Community Blood Centers, "Acquired Immune Deficiency Syndrome (AIDS) and Blood Transfusion".

1-4-84 Memorandum: Joseph Bove to Transfusion-Transmitted Diseases Committee Members, AABB. Re: CDC Update, Transfusion Associated AIDS, Conference Call, January 4, 1984.

1-9-84 AABB News release: "AABB Terms Risk of Transfusion-Associated AIDS 'extremely low'."

1-10-84 Internal Memorandum: Gerald Sandler to Alfred Katz, ARC. Re: Draft Paper Rationale for Anti-HBc Test.

1-10-84 Minutes: Scientific Advisory Committee, Irwin Memorial Blood Bank.

1-12-84 News release: American Red Cross, Blood Services, Central California Region, "CDC Study Shows Blood Donor Screening Procedures Work".

1-23-84 Memorandum: Roger Dodd to Gerald Sandler, ARC. Re: Rationale for anti-HBc testing of blood donors.

1-24-84 Medical Bulletin #10, Chapter Advisory #13: "NHF reaffirms position that product withdrawal should not change use of clotting factors.

1-30-84 Minutes: American Association of Blood Banks Meeting

1-30-84 Medical Bulletin #11: "Addressing Issues Concerning Hemophilia and the Potential Sexual Transmission of AIDS". Attachment: Chapter Advisory #14: "Questions Raised About Sexual Relations and AIDS."

1-30-84 Newsletter: AABB NewsBriefs.

2-6-84 Internal Memorandum: Brian McDonough to Hospital Administrators, Directors of Clinical Laboratories and Supervisors of Transfusion Services, Irwin Memorial Blood Bank.

2-8-84 Chart: TA-AIDS reported to CDC June 1981—February 8, 1984; Donor Investigations.

2-9-84 Presentation: "Current Strategies for the Identification and Exclusion of High Risk Donors" by John C. Petricciani, M.D. National Center for Drugs and Biologics Food and Drug Administration, Joint Meeting of Blood Products and Viral Products, U.K.

2-10-84 Newsletter: Council of Community Blood Centers.

2-17-84 Memorandum: Joseph Bove to Members of the Transfusion-Transmitted Diseases Committee. Re: AIDS Update.

2-17-84 Memo: Roger Dodd to Paul Cumming re: tests for AIDS

2-22-84 Memorandum: James W. Curran to Director, Center for Infectious Diseases. Re: Summary of February 14, 1984, Meeting on AIDS Related to Transfusions.

3-6-84 Final Report: Hepatitis B Core Anti-body Study Group

3-12-84 Letter: Peter Page to Alfred Katz, ARC.

3-13-84 Memorandum: John Hink to Distribution List. Re: Report on Hepatitis B Core Antibody Testing Study Group.

3-22-84 Letter: Dr. Luis Fajardo to "Director" ARC San Jose

3-29-84 Letter: Dr. Pearl Toy, ARC San Jose to Gerald Sandler

4-3-84 Letter: Dr. Alfred Katz to Dr. Pearl Toy

4-16-84 Letter: Lauren O'Brien, ARC San Jose to Dr. Alfred Katz

5-23-84 Minutes: Medical Advisory Committee Meeting

10-9-84 Internal Memo: Shelly Jordan to Nursing Staff, ARC. Attachment: Pamphlet, "New, Critical Information for Blood Donors."

10-13-84 NHF Medical Bulletin #15, Chapter Advisory #20, "Recommendations Concerning AIDS and the Treatment of Hemophilia".

11-5-84 NHF Medical Bulletin #17, Chapter Advisory #22, "Misleading information in edited press report stirs concern."

11-5-84 NHF Medical Bulletin #16, Chapter Advisory #21: "CDC Issues Update on AIDS and Hemophilia."

11-12-84 Newsletter: AABB News Briefs.

11-6-84 Minutes: FDA Blood Products Advisory Meeting.

12-10-84 Joint Statement: AABB, ARC and CCBC, "Transfusion-Associated AIDS: Interim Recommendations for Notification of Blood Collecting Organizations and Transfusion Services".

12-11-84   NHF Medical Bulletin #19: "AIDS Cases and Surveillance".

12-12-84   NHF Medical Bulletin #18, Chapter Advisory #23, "Heat Treated Factor IX Concentrate Now Available."

12-13-84   NHF Medical Bulletin #20, Chapter Advisory #24, "NHF reaffirms position that product withdrawal should not change use of clotting factor."

12-14-84   FDA Memorandum: Elaine Esber to All Establishments Collecting Blood, Blood Components or Source Plasma and all Licensed Manufacturers of Plasma Derivatives. Re: Revised Recommendations to Decrease the Risk of Transmitting Acquired Immunodeficiency Syndrome (AIDS) from Blood and Plasma Donors.

4-22-85   Memo: Dr. Julian Schorr to All Regional Blood Centers re: HTLV III antibody test results

5-28-85   Note: David Maserang, Abbott Labs to Dr. Fred Darr

6-6-86   Letter: W.T. Stall, Abbott Labs to Kay Ennis, ARC re: Red Cross Center test problems

6-18-86   Western Union Telegram: Bill Conrad, Abbott Labs to Medical Director, Syracuse Region ARC re: FDA approval

7-86   Lab Results: Genetic Systems test results to Roger Dodd

7-7-86   Conference Statement: NIH Consensus Development Conference re: HTLV III antibody test

8-6-86   Letter: Peter Tomasulo to Dr. James Landmark, Center Directors Council re: HTLV III test

11-1-86   Minutes: Center Directors Council

11-11-86   Memo: Victor Schmitt to Directors and Medical Directors, all ARC regional blood services

12-22-86   Minutes: Center Directors Council

12-24-86   Note: Victor Schmitt and Gerald Sandler to Peter Tomasulo, South Florida Region, Miami re: Abbott test delay

1-9-87   Memo: Dr. James Aubuchon, ARC to Directors, Scientific and Medical Directors, Center Chapter Managers

1-16-87   Memo: Dr. Sandler to all regional blood services, including Puerto Rico re: FDA approval

2-18-87   Memo: Delores Mallory, ARC to Task Force re: Infectious Disease test kits

1-15-92   Letter: Congressman John Dingell, Subcommittee on Oversights and Investigations to Elizabeth Dole

2-6-92   Letter: Mark E. Barmak, General Counsel Abbott Labs to Honorable John Dingell

5-19-94   Conference Agenda: Blood Services

5-24-94   Internal Newsletter: ARC Focus Magazine

7-8-94   Role and Responsibilities: Regional blood services board task force

8-5-94   Report: Regional Blood Services board task force

8-24-94   Memo: Pat Powers to Blood Services board re: task force activities

9-7-94   Agenda: Biomedical Service Board

10-7-94   Memo: Jimmy Ross and Brian McDonough to Senior Principal Officers and Principal Officers re: Biomedical cash flow conservation measures

10-24-94   Letter: Dr. William Swallow to Richard McFerson, CEO Nationwide Insurance re: Executive committee meeting of Board of Directors of NE Penn.

10-25-94   Memo: Jimmy Ross and Brian McDonough to Senior Principal Officers and Principal Officers re: strategies for cash flow maximization

4-24-95   Sharon Ritter-Smith and Jim Ross to Chapter Chairmen and Managers, Principal Officers, Regional Board Chairman re: Joint Biomedical Services and Chapter Cross Link

6-5-95   Letter: Dr. Ron Gilcher, President/CEO, Oklahoma

Blood Institute to Roy Clason, V.P., Communications, the Red Cross

10-95 Sales and Marketing Report: Red Cross Advantage: Focus on Safety Program

10-95 Financial Review: Budget Execution in process

12-1-95 ARC Biomedical Information Systems: Implementation and Support Organization

1995 Press Release and Packet: ARC New Independent Affiliate Program

1-16-96 Press Release: ARC Service in Memphis

2-15-96 Memo: Jimmy Ross to Senior Principal Officers, Principal Officers, Regional Board Chairmen and all Staff Directors re: plasma revenues

2-15-96 Bulletin: Executive special bulletin, Jenna Dorn re: Board of Governors Region-Chapter Issues, ARC Leadership Corner re: marketing

2-23-96 Minutes: Biomedical Services Board

3&4-96 Resolution III: Improving Regional and Chapter Relations

4-30-96 Memo: Norman Augustine, Gene Dyson to Chapter

INDEX